ACC

EMERGENCY MANUAL.

BY

W. A. YINGLING, M.D., Ph.D.,

MEMBER OF THE INTERNATIONAL HAHNEMANNIAN
ASSOCIATION.

---

*Haud facilem esse viam voluit, primusque per
Movit agros, curis acuens mortalia corda.*

VIRGIL.

B. Jain Publishers Pvt. Ltd.
New Delhi (India)

Price: Rs. 50.00

Reprint Edition : **2002**
© Copyright with the Publisher
Published by :
B. Jain Publishers Pvt. Ltd.
1921, Street No. 10, Chuna Mandi
Paharganj, New Delhi - 110 055 (INDIA)
Phones : 3683200, 3683300, 3670430, 3670572
FAX : 011-3683400 & 3610471
Email : bjain@vsnl.com
Website : www.bjainindia.com

Printed in India by :
Unisons Techno Financial Consultants (P) Ltd.
522, FIE, Patpar Ganj, Delhi - 110092.
ISBN 81-7021-329-0
BOOK CODE B-2563

PREFACE

the ... ... parturition of the bed

PREFACE.

NECESSITY is not only the mother of in-
vention, but the impelling force in the pre-
paration of such monographs as this little
book. Who, with a heart, does not pity the
suffering parturient woman; who would not
labor to relieve her sufferings when he felt
that he could. This has been the force behind the pen of the author. There need be
no excuse for sympathy.

Having relieved suffering, and hastened
to natural labor, cases that would otherwise
have been of necessity instrumental, by the
aid of the manuscript of this book, and
knowing from experience that the indicated
remedy is the parturient woman's best friend,
restoring the parts to a normal condition,
and giving as nearly a painless labor as the
circumstances and formation of the parts
permit, my sympathy for those who bring
into the world human life and the immortal

soul has induced me to offer this aid to the profession.

It is hoped this manual will lead the accoucheur to the indicated remedy direct, without hesitation or delay. The set of Repertories will aid in this. The experience of the many is that of uncertainty at the bedside, with the necessity of guessing or of returning to the office to "look up" the case, thus losing valuable time, or recourse to that worse practice of "regular" means and meddlesome midwifery. This manual will remedy this difficulty, and give the prescriber the power to relieve suffering, and bring glory to the great cause of Homœopathy. If the prescriber will depend on his remedies, carefully selecting them *at the bedside*, he will gain confidence in them and in himself, for in no sphere do the remedies act more promptly and efficiently, like magic transferring real *pain* into the expulsive force of labor without undue suffering.

Whilst all irregularities of labor cases can be controlled by the remedy alone, it will not enlarge the bony structure nor remove malformations congenital or induced by the manner of living; nor will it instantaneously remove the effects of local morbid growths, cancer, etc. Common sense discrimination must be exercised. The cases without the sphere of action of the homœopathic remedy are comparatively few. We have a universal law, and in no class of cases will the prescriber get better or quicker results than in those of labor. These are the reasons for this manual. Overlook the imperfections of detail and plan, and seek the good for the relief of your trusting and expectant patient.

W. A. YINGLING.

INTRODUCTION

THE object of this Manual is to give assistance in the emergency, at the bedside, and to preclude the necessity of carrying one or more large volumes as aids, or of going to the office for help. It is presumed that the user is fully acquainted with all the various presentations, the irregularities of the parts, the use of instruments, the manner of turning, etc., etc.

This work deals exclusively with the remedies and their application to the abnormal conditions of parturition, those which occur directly before, during, or after labor or abortion. It does not deal with those conditions wherein the physician has plenty of time for consideration, as in many ailments during gestation, and those following some days after delivery. It is strictly an emergency manual, yet containing all the symptoms of the rubrics treated of, and many indications of remedies not usually consid-

ered critical, as it is impossible to tell beforehand what symptoms may be the keynotes
in the emergency hour to either save life or
prevent undue suffering. Strictly speaking,
only those conditions endangering life would
be emergency conditions, but as any undue
suffering or abnormality may be the pre-
cursor or direct cause of the emergency condition, indications of remedies covering these
must, of necessity, be included in such a
work. As far as possible, all indications of
remedies for labor and abortion, with hæmorrhage and eclampsia, are given.

In the urgent desire to have *all* the symptoms that might be possibly called for in the
emergency, and to give a true picture of the
remedy, some symptoms which may seem
far-fetched are included. It is by far safer
to have a few symptoms that may never or
seldom be used, than to omit any that might
save life or suffering. Then, in the homœopathic treatment of any case it is impossible
to tell what symptom may be indicative of
the simillimum, or what remedy may be
called for. Any remedy in the whole range
of homœopathic materia medica may be
indicated in any given case. The patient in

hand must be treated, and the symptoms alone must point to the curative remedy. This rule must hold good in obstetrical practice as in any other: *Give the remedy the pathogenesis of which entirely covers the symptoms of the patient*, even though it has never been used or even thought of in connection with such a case or condition. From this fact some remedies may be unwittingly omitted, but not to any great extent it is hoped.

The plan of the work is simple. The first part contains the therapeutic indications of the remedies under the various rubrics. Whilst the rubrics are distinct in their general features, yet the peculiarity of the given remedy may be consulted by taking the therapeutics as a whole. The repetition of symptoms under the various rubrics is intended to impress upon the attention of the prescriber those red-string peculiarities that will generally be found present when the remedy is called for. In the Generalities we endeavor to give a bird's eye view of each remedy so as to enable the prescriber to decide definitely in case of doubt. Definite pictures are presented of each remedy which, if the eye focuses aright, will aid materially in selecting the true simillimum.

Whilst the rubric Abortion is quite complete, yet it will be well to consult, as symptoms indicate, the rubrics Labor, Hæmorrhage, and Retained Placenta. For symptoms other than the character of the flow in hæmorrhage, the other rubrics may also be consulted. So with convulsions. Thus the rubrics are interchangeable to a certain extent. All symptoms are of the patient, nature calling for a remedy, and not from the *name* of the sickness; hence, a general symptom may be applicable to all diseases and conditions.

We place hour-glass contractions under Labor, as these may occur during labor as well as with retained placenta, or at any time.

Under Hæmorrhage we give a few symptoms for menorrhagia as they are of such a character as to be useful in puerperal metrorrhagia.

The repertories are as complete as needful. References are made in each to others as required by the demands of the case. A careful study of them will facilitate greatly the search for a remedy in an emergency.

To be useful, a tool must be understood. It is poor policy, and usually the cause of objection, to learn the use of a help in the hour of greatest need. To be familiar with the help is about one-half of the time and labor required to utilize it. To familiarize oneself with the repertories, it is well to take various symptoms at random, and look them up in the repertories, noting any peculiarity of the author's mind in placing them. References can be added by the researcher for future assistance. This suggestion is applicable to those who are unfamiliar with the use of repertories.

There are but few symptoms to be given under the rubric "The Baby," but we arrange them in a separate repertory for the convenience of those who may use this manual.

We have not the space to give any lengthy dissertation on several very important questions pertaining to homœopathic prescribing, but there are several things we want to say, at least to call attention to them, and, if possible, to inspire confidence in those who are wavering in their faith and practice.

Will homœopathy produce natural labor? We answer, it is the *only* means whereby abnormal labor may be made as natural as the condition and circumstance will permit. Whilst it will not change the bony structure, it will restore the soft parts to a normal condition unless prevented by local disease, like cancer or cicatrices, and even with these it will reduce the suffering to the minimum. It will relieve suffering and produce normal uterine contractions, and enable the parturient woman to cheerfully bear the ordeal as no other means is capable of doing. Back of the condition, back of the state of the parts is the nervous system, the vital force, and the cause of the derangement, either of which is reached and controlled by the homœopathic remedy. It is wonderful, magical indeed, to observe the rapid action of the simillimum in obstetrical practice.

Where the wise physician has charge of his patient during the months of gestation normal labor, labor without undue suffering, may be induced. Homœopathy is the woman's best friend. It is the only means whereby she may procreate with the minimum of suffering. It is the only means whereby normal labor, with all that that term implies, can be certainly .secured.

This, of course, is applicable to those cases where the bony structure is not misshapen or the soft parts made undilatable by local disease. Even these may be somewhat controlled by timely treatment, on the principle that a "stitch in time saves nine." By the use of pure homœopathy the vast majority of cases resulting in loss of life or in excruciating suffering from the supposed irregularities of the parts would terminate happily and easily. All that is needed is confidence and knowledge on the part of the attending physician. The people are willing and anxious to be led. The people have more confidence in the powers of homœopathy than many are willing to allow. They follow implicitly the direction of their allopathic attendant in hopes of relief. They *would* follow as implicitly the advice of their homœopathic attendant if he would manifest confidence in his system of medicine and insist upon obedience, with the positive result of a most favorable consummation; so favorable that the glad tidings would go from woman to woman with the celerity of happy news, resulting in the rapid spread of the glad tidings of pure homœopathy. If I am an enthusiast on this subject it results from what I have seen with my own eyes, and the result of the course I have herein advocated and advised. Let the physician be true to homœopathy, and I assure him homœopathy will never fail him in an emergency.

The only direction that can be given for prescribing is to follow the direction of Samuel Hahnemann as given in *The Organon* and *The Chronic Diseases.* Discard every fad, every allopathic adjunct, and rely implicitly on the homœopathic remedy. Live or die true to your declared principles. The female eunuchs, female invalids, and female maniacs, resulting directly from allopathic means of meddlesome midwifery, should deter any follower of Hahnemann from resorting to their means of treatment. It is poor policy to follow the lead of blind guides, mariners without a chart or compass upon the great sea of medicine, simply groping their way from fad to fad, from theory to theory, in hopes of finding the panacea applicable to a name or condition of disease.

The homœopathician has not much use for the forceps and other obstetrical instru-

ments, and yet he should always be prepared to use them in cases of *real* necessity.
I would advise, however, that the remedy
be given a fair trial first, and that the instruments be the last resort. By this means
their aid will be very seldom needed. I
make no complaint against the instruments,
as they are sometimes necessary, but I pro-
test against their indiscriminate and hasty
use, frequently to the detriment of the mother
and child.

The course herein advised will also prevent the rupture of the perinæum in the
very great majority of cases. There is no
need to tear a woman to pieces. It may be
scientific, but it is not rational nor homœopathic. The Creator did not produce the
soft parts of woman for the purpose of ex-
hibiting the skill of the gynæcologist. That
is the result of the wilful ignorance and
haste of the accoucheur. "The human
perinæum has in like manner been adapted
to its office . . . . My contention is this:
Laceration of the perinæum should be of
very rare occurence. It is a contradiction
of all we know in regard to the process of
nature to claim that she cannot make a peri-

næum that is able to stand the stress and
strain which any natural use can put upon
it."*

I do not believe in the use of chloroform
in labor, except in extreme cases where
the simillimum cannot be found or where instruments are necessary. It precludes the
proper administration of the homœopathic
remedy, which we deem so essential and
efficient. "The immense power dependent
upon the action of the muscles of the woman,
apart from those of the uterus, is more or
less dependent on the will, and hence, it will
be perceived, the use of chloroform must
interfere with labor to the extent that it
lessens the power to cause voluntary muscular efforts."†

"It seems merciful to relieve this great
suffering promptly with chloroform, but it
is more merciful to relieve it in the only
right way by the homœopathic remedy when
it is possible, because the relief is a real one
and beneficial in its effect on the whole

---

* G. W. Winterburn, M.D., in *Med. Advance*, xxix.,
p. 89.

† Guernsey, *Obstet.*, p. 179.

case, instead of merely palliating the pain."*
" If enough Ether be given to relax the perinæum, then labor is going to stop,† and so
deep anæsthesia is very apt to injure the
child. Another point to consider is that post-
partum hæmorrhage is likely to follow."‡
" A woman is more susceptible during labor
and pregnancy to the action of remedies than
at any other time. . . . . An anæsthetic
masks symptoms, prolongs suffering in the
end, increases the liability to hæmorrhage,
to mastitis, and other troubles of the mam-
mary glands. . . . . Keep to the indicated
remedy; it does as much for both mother
and child during labor as it does during the
`dynamics of gestation."§ It is claimed that
some women *demand* an anæsthetic. Who
is to do the prescribing, the doctor or the
woman? She is simply following a custom,
and *knows no better.* No physician with manhood will permit his patient to dictate his

---

* Dr. J. T. Kent, *Hom. Physician*, xi., p. 96.

† In many women I have seen labor entirely cease
from even partial anæsthesia, but these are the excep-
tion.—Burt's *Materia Medica*, p. 274.

‡ Dr. J. B. Bell, *Hom. Physician*, xi., p. 97.

§ Dr. H. C. Allen, *Ibid.*

2

treatment. Herein is the reason of disrespect shown to the homœopathic physician; he allows allopathic notions to dictate his procedure and prescription. Would an allopath of honor allow his patient to dictate homœopathic treatment? If the patient desires a homœopath to treat her, let her receive pure homœopathic treatment. As soon as the people learn that the homœopathic profession has the righteous determination to assert its rights and insist on submission to homœopathic practices and means, they will respect the profession and gracefully submit. In the end this course will bring both honor and riches. A physician has more to do than to *keep his patients* and make money. He must respect his own manhood and the honor of his profession. The people will not respect a man who does not respect himself.

Neither do I believe in the antiseptic injections following labor. Preventive medicine is right and proper in its place, if homœopathic, but it is the height of folly to use it in imaginary troubles. The physician should know whether there is danger of septic poisoning, and if he have symptoms pointing that way, the very best thing for him to do is to give the indicated homœopathic remedy which will correct matters speedily. There is positively no danger from the lochial discharge in the healthy woman. If she is not healthy there will be present symptoms in her or her discharge pointing to the proper homœopathic remedy. This is another allopathic fad causing harm, and hence is worse than useless. I have been present where confinement took place in a dug-out of one small room, which was used for every purpose of the family; where the floor was the mother earth covered with pools of dish water and besmeared with disgusting expectoration; where bed bugs were an active army, and the bedding was so dirty that I was most anxious to strain my back to prevent contact; where I was disgusted with odors and distressed with hunger; and yet, *without vaginal injections*, the woman was free from all untoward conditions, was up and doing her own work in ten days, and performing the full functions of a *wife*. I have attended others nearly as bad without evil results. If the preventive treatment were essential at all, surely it would be in such cases. The only remaining question arises, are the clean, **pure** women of fashionable society dirtier within than the many of the hovels? I answer most emphatically, No. The trouble is with the physician and not with the works of nature.

In placenta prævia I fully recommend the method or plan of Dr. H. N. Guernsey, which is "*in puncturing the membranes through the placenta and evacuating the liquor amnii.*" "The finger must explore a sulcus between the cotyledons of the placenta, and with the same hand a female catheter, previously concealed in the palm, must be forced through the placenta and the membranes during a pain." "The liquor amnii *must be drawn off slowly*: and as surely as it thus flows, so surely will the hæmorrhage cease. After the waters have pretty much escaped, the finger may take the place of the catheter, and aid in tearing the orifice larger, so that the presenting parts may descend." This method applies whether the placenta is central or only partially over the os uteri.

In no class of cases will the homœopathic remedy be found to act more efficiently and speedily than in post-partum hæmorrhage.

It is really astonishing how rapidly a profuse hæmorrhage will cease after the administration of the properly selected simillimum. Here the adjuncts and appliances of the "regular" system are more than useless. The physician should be prepared to select the remedy speedily, but time will be saved to carefully get all the symptoms, and as carefully to select the remedy. When the simillimum is administered the hæmorrhage will cease in a very short time, or at least be under control, so as not to endanger the life of the woman. In such emergency cases nature speaks plainly. The more danger to life the more plainly nature speaks. And in like manner, *the more danger to life the more speedily will the homœopathic remedy act.* This is a fact corroborated by the experience of the best prescribers. Only those who trust to the well-selected remedy are safe from calamity in such cases. The symptoms present during the progress of labor will very often point to the remedy to be used in hæmorrhage, or if given in time will prevent it. The physician should be fortified against an emergency by anticipating trouble. In most instances he can read over the repertories and refresh his memory whilst waiting the progress of the case. Time thus spent will give better returns than the gossip of the lying-in chamber.

The same remarks apply to puerperal eclampsia. Homœopathy in the hands of the cool and self-possessed is supreme and always reliable in these trying cases. The stampeded and weak will forsake his only sheet-anchor, and rush to the appliances of the regulars for very questionable assistance. Our only hope is in being true to our calling as homœopathic physicians. Try it fairly, and every one will become an enthusiast for the true science of therapeutics.

We feel constrained to write a few words in regard to the potency and the repetition of the dose. Every one acknowledges that the low potencies act, and at times most brilliantly. There is no difference in regard to this. But those who have fairly tried the higher potencies are just as sure, and from the same reason, that of experience, that they act much more promptly and efficiently, and in many cases will cure where the low entirely fail. From actual experience we sincerely assert that the higher potencies are by far the best to use in labor cases, especially, and that their best and quickest action is seen in the most alarming emergency cases. We have seen the most profuse hæmorrhage cease in a very few moments after the exibition of a single dose of a high potency. We have seen the most distressing pains change like magic into genuine labor-pains, with delivery following speedily and naturally after a high potency. My own experience with high potencies has been so satisfactory and gratifying that I feel it a duty to urge every user of this manual to give them a fair trial. Select the remedy carefully, and the speedy result will be to make another enthusiast in favor of the highly potentized remedies.

In emergency cases the action of the simillimum is so speedy that there is seldom need for a repetition of the dose, if of a high potency. If there is no change following the administration, it shows that the wrong remedy has been given, and another must be selected. The length of time to wait on the action of the remedy must be determined by the judgment of the physician, and the demands of the emergency. In the ordinary complaints of labor it is well to wait an half hour, whereas, in alarming hæmorrhage, but a few moments. If no result follows, a new remedy must be selected. If there is a change for the better, the only rational act is to wait until there is need for a repetition of the same remedy, or until the symptoms point to another. No rule can be laid down to govern the decision of the prescriber. It all depends on his selection of the remedy, and the case in hand. Yet it is safe to say that after a careful selection of a remedy it is best to wait its action a reasonable time— the emergency must decide that—and not to repeat the dose or change the remedy without a plain and sufficient reason. If there is improvement, it would be folly to repeat or change as long as that improvement is decided and continuous. If there is no change for the better within the reasonable time as above, it would be folly to wait longer. This applies especially to the use of the high potencies. Whilst it is always wisest to take time to select the proper remedy, yet we know that the mass of prescribers frequently fail in their first attempt, even when careful. In such a case we do not esteem it detrimental to the case to change to another remedy as soon as the mistake is discovered, or even to make several such changes, especially where there has not been frequent and rapid repetition, such as would produce a proving of the drug. With the high potencies these frequent repetitions are unnecessary, as the true simillimum will act promptly in all these complaints of the parturient woman, and it will be easy to tell whether the proper remedy has been selected.

PART I.

THERAPEUTIC INDICATIONS.

PART I.

THERAPEUTIC INDICATIONS.

ACETICUM ACIDUM.

Labor:

HÆMORRHAGE.—*After labor*. With coldness, pallor, and difficult breathing. *With great thirst*, not relieved by drinking. Active or passive. (Outward application of vinegar to the vulva is also advised when indicated.)

GENERALITIES.—Anxiousness. Sadness. Fearful of persons and surroundings. Irritable. Delirium, alternating with unconsciousness. Head heavy, hot, with distended temporal vessels. Cold sweat on forehead. Face emaciated, pale, waxen. Cheeks flushed and hot: Hissing respiration, with rattling in larynx and trachea. Burning thirst for large quantities of water. Thirst insatiable, not relieved by drinking. Pain in spine relieved by lying on the abdomen. Pale and waxen skin. Lax, lean, pale persons. Fainting. Hot flushes. Jumps from the bed and crawls on the floor, howling with pain. Great weakness. Dropsy, with great thirst.

ACONITUM.

Labor:

The vulva, vagina, and os are dry, tender, and undilatable; the parts feel contracted and rigid. Great distress, moaning, and *restlessness* with each pain (or after). She fears she will not be delivered, or that she will die, or that something will certainly go wrong. Cessation of the pain when the cause is akin to *fright.* Spasmodic contraction of the os, with heat and dryness. Intolerant of examination from local sensitiveness. Fainting. Full of anxiety and fear. Pains unnaturally violent and frequent; complains that she cannot breathe or bear the pains; hot sweat all over; contractions insufficient. Headache.

ABORTION.—From cystitis; from fright, with vexation; from fright when the fear remains, and she does not seem to get over it; from plethora; from anger. Fear that something terrible will happen to her; fear of death; dizzy on rising from a recumbent position; afraid to turn over, to move, or to leave the bed. Anxiety with great nervousness and excitability. Hæmorrhage predominating.

HÆMORRHAGE.—*Active*, with fear of death, moving, turning, or of something to happen. Very giddy; she cannot sit up in bed or rise up. Excitement. *Plethoric, dark-haired young women.* From fright. Is sure she will die.

CONVULSIONS.—Hot, dry skin, thirst, restlessness, fear of death, cerebral congestion; numbness and tingling of the limbs. In *primiparæ*, with spasms of os, and with the foregoing symptoms at the commencement of labor, especially :

AFTER-PAINS.—Painful and strong; too long lasting.

THE BABY.—Asphyxia, apoplectic symptoms, hot, purplish, breathless, pulseless, or nearly so; icterus; ophthalmia; *retained urine.*

GENERALITIES.— *Violent palpitation of the heart;* congestion of blood to the head; buzzing in the ears; pale face on rising up; *after a fright;* fear of death, predicts the day;

anxiety inconsolable, piteous wailing; reproaches others for mere trifles; peevish, impatient; restless, agonized tossing about. Oversensitive, cannot bear light or noise; will not be touched or uncovered. Fainting on rising from a recumbent position, with pale face or congestion to the head. Great thirst. Sensation as if the whole brain would be pressed out at the forehead.

ALETRIS FARINOSA.

ABORTION.—*Habitual* tendency to abortion in feeble persons of lax fibre and anæmic condition, even after hæmorrhage has set in; weight in uterine region, tendency to prolapsus uteri; general weakness of mind and body; weak from long sickness or defective nutrition or loss of fluids. Dyspepsia.

HÆMORRHAGE.—Passive. Menorrhagia, profuse, black blood and coagula; fulness and weight in the uterine region.

AMYL NITRITE

Labor:

Spasmodic pains and contraction of the os uteri; flushing with each pain and severe headache. *Very painful* labor from a spasmodically constricted os.

CONVULSIONS.—Immediately after delivery, with intense rushing of blood to the face and head in paroxysms, making them red and hot. Rapid succession of spasms. Muscles become rigid. Piercing shrieks.

GENERALITIES.—Cannot endure warmth, must throw off all covering, and open the doors and windows, even in cold weather. Heat, throbbing and intense fulness in the head. The head is heavy, giddy, and confused with prostration. Protruding, staring eyes, and look as if glazed, in convulsions. Throbbing in ears. Sense of constriction in throat, which extends to the chest. Difficulty in breathing.

ANTIMONIUM CRUDUM.

HÆMORRHAGE.—Uterine, with distinct pressure in the womb, as if something would come out. Somewhat rheumatic.

GENERALITIES.—*White tongue;* nausea and vomiting. Fretful, peevish, *dislikes to be looked at or touched.* Great sadness and woeful mood. Sulky, does not wish to speak to any one.

ANTIMONIUM TARTARICUM.

Labor :

Rigid os uteri with much nausea and dyspnœa, especially in women with a history of subacute or chronic pelvic inflammations.

CONVULSIONS.—After the child is born. Convulsive twitching in almost every muscle of the face.

THE BABY.—Apparent death ; rattling of mucus in the throat ; pale, gasping, breathless, although the cord still feebly pulsates. Suffocative form.

GENERALITIES.—Trembling of the head and hands. Pitiful whining and crying. Complains much ; despair of recovery. Dizzy when lifting the head from the pillow. Face a picture of anxiety and despair. Much mucus in the throat, rattling. Rapid, short, difficult and anxious respiration. Irritable. Much yawning and stretching. Drowsiness. Prostration.

APIS MELLIFICA.

Labor :

ABORTION.—From constipation ; from plethora. In the early months ; second month ;

third and fourth months, with profuse flow. Labor-like pains in the uterine region, extending into the thighs. Pain predominates. Stinging pain in one or the other ovarian region more and more frequent till labor-pains are produced; followed by pain and flow. *Urine scanty* (or profuse). No thirst. Prolonged and difficult constipation. Restlessness. Yawning.

HÆMORRHAGE.—Active. Dark. Profuse, with heaviness in the abdomen; faintness. Great uneasiness, and yawning. Red spots like bee-stings on the skin, and stinging sensation in the ovarian region and elsewhere. Brought on or sustained by hatred or jealousy. Restlessness.

CONVULSIONS.—Drowsiness; scanty urine, high-colored and albuminous. Twitching; trembling; jactitation of muscles. With convulsive laughter.

GENERALITIES.—*Pains like bee-stings*. Absence of thirst. Urine scanty. Great tearfulness, cannot help crying. Irritable. Fidgety. Nothing seems to satisfy. Restlessness. Yawning. Great sensitiveness to touch or light pressure. *Tired, as if bruised all over*. Lassitude. Loss of consciousness.

Sopor interrupted by piercing shrieks. Muttering delirium. Dread of death. Confused vertigo, worse sitting, extreme when lying and closing the eyes; nausea and headache. General feeling of suffocation.

APOCYNUM CANNABINUM.

HÆMORRHAGE.—Continuous or in paroxysms. Profuse. Fluid, or in large clots or shreds. Great irritability of the stomach. *Urinary and dropsical complications.* Nausea, vomiting, palpitation; pulse quick, feeble, when moved; fainting when raised from the pillow. Brown flux.

GENERALITIES.—Bewildered, low-spirited, stupid. Face bloated, worse lying down. Sense of general, but transient debility.

ARGENTUM NITRICUM.

ABORTION.—Disposed to abortion.

HÆMORRHAGE.—Confusion, dulness and pain in the head, aggravated by the least movement. *A short time seems very long to her.* Everything done seems done too slowly. Belching wind relieves her distress. Worse from motion.

CONVULSIONS.—She has a presentiment of

the coming spasm. The stomach feels as if it would burst with wind, with marked relief of all symptoms after belching, which comes up in a torrent. She is in constant motion during the interval between spasms, tossing about from side to side; or she may lie quiet for a while, and then become very restless before another sets in. Spasms are violent, and are preceded by *a sensation of general expansion* of the whole body, but especially of the face and head.

THE BABY.—Ophthalmia, profuse, purulent discharge.

GENERALITIES.—Apathy. Taciturn and gloomy. Time passes too slowly; it seems as if others were very slow in doing things for her. Easily excited, nervous, irritable, anxious. Headache, better by being bound up tightly. Vertigo as if turning in a circle. Longing for sugar. Noisy belching, with general relief. Sensation of a splinter in the throat, or in various parts. Debility, especially of the legs and calves of legs. Faint feeling. Almost constant belching of wind after eating, which continues nearly to the next meal. Pains in the back and lower extremities.

ARNICA MONTANA.

Labor:

Fatigue of uterus, causing too feeble or irregular pains, with a sense of weariness. Flushed face and heat of the head with the pains, while the rest of the body may be cool. The pains accomplish but little, though they are so violent as to drive her almost to distraction. Pains distressing. False pains. She *feels sore and bruised* in any position, and must often change position. Fainting from injuries, from fatigue, or from stitches about the heart. *Head hot and body cool.* Intolerant of examination from local sensitiveness. Feeble pains, with constant desire to change position. Great soreness of back during labor, with too great sensitiveness to pain. Labor pains weak and ceasing. Soreness apparently resulting from abnormal sensitiveness of the neck of the uterus to the pressure of the child's head.

ABORTION.—*From a fall, a shock, a bruise, or concussion.* Flowing without pain, pain without flow, or both pain and flow. She feels bruised and sore; it hurts her to move; the child hurts her when it moves (when far enough along to have motion). The child feels as if it laid crosswise in the abdomen. Pain predominates. Bed feels too hard. Discharge is continuous, profuse, bright red, coagulated, or serous mucus. Pain in the uterine region, labor-like, from urging. Threatened septicæmia after abortion. (*Pyrogen.*)

HÆMORRHAGE.—From fatigue, concussion, or shock. Constant bright red or clotted flux, with or without pain. Nausea at pit of stomach. Head hot and body cool. *She feels sore, as if bruised in the uterine region.* Active. Bright red, with large clots or lumpy. From traumatism; protracted labors; instrumental deliveries. " Womb wide open, profuse *pale* blood mixed with *large black clots.*" (Clinical.)

RETAINED PLACENTA.—

CONVULSIONS.—Head hot and body cool or of a natural temperature. Full, strong pulse, and during every pain the blood rushes violently to the face and head. Symptoms of *paralysis of the left side.* Loss of consciousness. Involuntary stool and urine. Abdominal tympanitis after labor.

AFTER-PAINS.—*Arnica* (high) will often entirely prevent after-pains when administered at close of labor (unless contra-indicated) that has been bruising to the parts and straining to the general muscular system. Pains violent. It aids in restoring the parts to their natural condition. *Pains excited by nursing the baby.*

THE BABY.—Traumatic tetanus; face hot, body cold; jerking breathing; tremor of limbs. *Asphyxia.*

GENERALITIES.—Bad effects of mechanical injuries. Head hot, body cool. *Bruised* sensation in any part of the body. Sensation as of a concussion, as from a fall. Hopeless. Peevish. Sensitive. Indifference. Quarrelsome. Thoughtless gaiety ; great frivolity and mischievousness. Eructations tasting of hard-boiled eggs. Retention of the urine, which is painful. Black-and-blue spots on the body. Fears being struck or touched by persons coming near her. Twitching of the muscles. *Great sinking of strength.* Bed feels too hard. The motions of the fœtus cause a bruised and sore feeling in the abdomen, and the child seems to lie crosswise, which position causes constant pain ; soreness in the symphysis pubis or in the sacro-iliac symphyses prevent her moving about during pregnancy without pain and discomfort.

ARSENICUM ALBUM.

Labor:

Debility or prostration when the least effort causes fainting. Thirst for frequent sips of cold water. Chilly, desires to be wrapped up warmly. Pale bloating of the face. A sense of great exhaustion after every effort, however small. Great restlessness and fear. Rigidity of the vagina and soft parts, so that they will hardly admit the index finger.

ABORTION.—See Generalities.

HÆMORRHAGE.—Lancinating and burning pains. Low state of the system when aphthæ appears. Dark, suddenly appearing.

CONVULSIONS.—General œdema; a waxy, puffy look of the face. Chilliness; extremities cold and clammy. Albuminuria; urine dark and scanty. Vomiting. Diarrhœa. Great thirst. Respiration short, difficult, anxious. Great prostration. Trembling of the hands. Each spasm is followed by great exhaustion and restlessness. Pale as if dead, though warm. Suddenly arouses and goes into severe convulsions, only again to relapse into a sort of cataleptic rigidity. Opisthotonos. Foam at mouth.

THE BABY.—Tetanic spasms, with frightful concussion of the limbs. Babe lies as if dead, pale but warm; breathless for some time; features distorted. Stiffness of limbs, particularly of the feet and knees. Skin dry like parchment.

GENERALITIES.—Great amount of *anguish*. Restlessness, anxious tossing and jerking about, every movement being followed by exhaustion. Exhaustion especially felt when moving; looks pale and haggard. Intense burning sensation. Fear of death; useless to do anything, as she surely will die. Delirium. Sad. Rapid sinking of strength. Stiffness of the limbs. Suffering often induces shuddering, coldness, anguish, prostration. Wants to be wrapped up warmly. Thirst for frequent small quantities of water. Expression of face anxious, but not wild. Respiration short and anxious. Palpitation of the heart, with anguish; cannot lie on back. Frequent fainting. Sense of warm air streaming up the spine into the head. Retention of urine after labor, with no sensation as of desire to urinate, though it is time it should pass. Periodical toothache during pregnancy, occurring mostly at night, driving patient almost to frenzy.

ASARUM EUROPÆUM.

Labor:

ABORTION.—Habitual tendency to abortion. Threatened from excessive sensibility of all the nerves; from even imagining something unpleasant might happen to her, a disagreeable sensation is felt, momentarily arresting all her thoughts and functions. Discharge black.

GENERALITIES.—Chilliness predominates; want of vital heat. Sensation as though all the body, or a part of the body, were being pressed together. *Great nervous irritation.* A feeling as if the body was hovering in the air. So sensitive and nervous that even thinking of the scratching of silk, or similar material, a thrill runs through her and aggravates all her symptoms. Tearing pain from the crest of one ilium to the other. Bruised pain in the back. General weary feeling.

ATROPINUM.

Labor:

CONVULSIONS.—After normal birth violent convulsions, unconsciousness: deep-red, distorted face; rolling eyes; gnashing teeth;

bloody foam before the mouth; bending in of thumbs; throwing about the limbs; on remission stretching of body and deep sopor.

AURUM METALLICUM.

Labor:

The pains make her desperate, so that she would like to jump out of the window and kill herself. Congestion to head and chest. Palpitation of heart. Irregularity in the pains, and when she rises up for anything, instead of lying down again quietly, she *thrashes herself down hard*.

GENERALITIES.—Great desire to commit suicide—to jump from the window or from a height. Desire for fresh air. Violent hysterics, accompanied with desperate actions. Anguish of mind and great grief; seems to have no friends. Looks on the dark side of everything; weeps and prays. Hopelessness and despondency, she has no confidence in herself, and thinks others have none. Mental irritability. Sad, feels that all is against her and life is not desirable, and the thought of death alone gives pleasure. Objects appear as if divided horizontally.

BELLADONNA.

Labor :

Pains come and go suddenly, with too quick bearing down, as if everything in the pelvis would be ejected; pains disappear suddenly. *Spasmodic contraction of the os,* which is hot, tender, red, and inclined to be somewhat moist (Acon., dry). Os uteri thin and rigid, more of a spasmodic contraction (Gels., thick and rigid). Labor slow and tedious, feels off and on only a pressure on sacrum. Pains violent and cause great distress, and yet the child does not advance. Pains cease; deficient. Drawing pains from the small of the back to thigh. Back feels as if it would break. Hot face, throbbing headache. Very red face, and eyes injected. Sensitive to noise, light, *jarring of the bed.* Primiparæ (pains suddenly cease). *Old maids in first delivery, muscles rigid.* Intolerant of examination from nervousness. Heat and tenderness of the parts. Swooning. False pains. The bed feels very hard to her. Hour-glass contractions. Moaning. Amniotic fluid gone, yet the os seems spasmodically contracted. Throbbing of the carotids. All her motions are quick.

ABORTION.—Violent aching and tensive pains through whole of body, with sensation of constriction and tension. Pains and discharge come suddenly and cease as suddenly. Pressing towards vulva, as if all internal organs would be pushed out. Pain in the back as if broken or would break. More or less discharge of blood which feels very hot. Cerebral congestion and moaning, which gives her temporary relief. Worse from least jar. Red face and eyes. Hæmorrhage predominates. Discharge coagulated; comes and goes suddenly; dark; offensive; bright red; hot; profuse; intermittent. Pain in the uterine region, colicky, labor-like. From uterine congestion. The least jar is unpleasant to her.

HÆMORRHAGE.—Profuse discharge of *bright red hot blood with downward pressure*, or forcing outward, as if everything would be forced out. Pain in the back as if it would break. Blood coagulates easily and is sometimes dark and offensive. *Flowing between the after-pains*. Hot, red face and head, congested eyes and full, bounding pulse. Aggravated from light, motion, noise, and *the least jar*. Large offensive clots. From fright. From retained placenta. After natural labor, especially.

RETAINED PLACENTA.—Red face and injected eyes. Great distress and moaning. *Heat and dryness of vagina.* Profuse flow of hot blood which speedily coagulates. Slightest jar causes suffering. Hour-glass contractions. Dryness and heat of surface.

CONVULSIONS.—Convulsive movements in the limbs and of the muscles of the face. Paralysis of *right side* of tongue. Loss of speech and difficult deglutition. Dilated pupils. Red or livid face. Renewal of spasms at every pain. Unconsciousness, or more or less tossing about between the spasms, or deep sleep, with grimaces or starts and cries, with fearful visions. Jerking and twitching of muscles between the spasms. Sound sleep or unconsciousness after a spasm. She appears as if stunned. Semi-consciousness. Foam at the mouth (may have a rotten odor). She may have a pale and cold face with shivering. Fixed or convulsive eyes. Involuntary escape of urine or fæces. Violent pulsations of the carotids. (The first remedy to think of.)

AFTER-PAINS.—Pains come and go very

quickly. Forcing pains, as if the contents of the pelvis would be forced through the vulva. Every jar hurts. *Lochial discharge feels hot.* Flow increased with every pain. She cannot endure noise, light or jar of the bed. Head and eyes congested.

THE BABY.—Asphyxia; apoplectic form; face very red, eyeballs injected, pupils dilated. Trismus with sudden starting and drawing together of body and limbs; anxious spasmodic respiration; motionless, staring eyes; inability to swallow, followed by spasms.

GENERALITIES.—Remarkable quickness of sensation, or of motion; the eyes snap and move quickly; pains come and go with great celerity; a pain may have lasted for some time, then in a second it is gone. Much twitching and jerking of the muscles. Delirious, with dulness; with raving and disposed to injure, strike, bite, etc. Moaning, which seems to relieve. Fantastic illusions, ghosts, hideous faces, black dogs, insects. She has a wild look, a stunned appearance. Throbbing and stitches. Boring head into pillow; constantly moving it from side to side. Face red; changing color frequently; very pale and suddenly red; distorted with pain. Plethora. Talkative, then mute. Quarrelsome, during exuberant mirth. Sensitive to noise, jar, etc. Redness of the eyes, with flushed face. Congestion of the sexual organs, with or without discharge of blood. Pain in the back, as if it would break. Frontal headache, with pressure and photophobia. The bed feels very hard. Objects appear dim; as if inverted or double. Ulcerative or throbbing toothache. "When *Bell.* is inefficient in a Belladonna case, give Lachesis." (Farrington.)

BORAX.

Labor:

Labor-pains dart upward, the child's head goes back. Pains spasmodic, more violent in stomach than in the uterus, accompanied by violent and frequent eructations. Pains too weak. Pains ceasing. False laborpains. She fears a downward motion. Very sensitive to any noise, as the rattling of paper or the door-latch, etc., etc.

GENERALITIES.—Great nervousness, easily startled by any noise. *Great fear of downward motion of any kind.* Anguish and fear.

Finds fault. Changeable. Breath smells mouldy. Taste of cellar mould when coughing. Very sensitive aptha, bleeding easily.

BRYONIA ALBA.

Labor:

Fainting from the least motion, even when no effort is required. Sighing respiration. Thirst for cold water in large quantities. Drawing or lancinating pains from hip to foot, worse from touch or motion.

ABORTION.—Discharge dark-red blood. From constipation; stool dry, as if burnt. Pain in back, worse from motion. Burning pain in uterus. Pain all over, extremities and all. Lips and mouth dry. Nausea on sitting up. Desires to be quiet. Splitting headache. Thirst for a large quantity of fluid.

HÆMORRHAGE.—Profuse. Dark fluid blood. *Dark red blood, with pain in the back, and a splitting headache. Dry mouth and lips; much thirst.* Nausea and faintness on sitting up, or even raising the head from the pillow. Increased by *the slightest movement of any part of the body,* even the head, or foot, or speaking.

CONVULSIONS.—She cannot bear to move or to be moved. After the spasms have been controlled, and there remain full hard pulse, thirst, abdominal tenderness, perspiration, and dry parched lips.

AFTER-PAINS.—*Excited by the least motion,* or even by taking a deep inspiration. She desires to lie perfectly quiet. Splitting headache. Parched lips and dry mouth and throat. Thirst for large quantity of cold water.

GENERALITIES.—She is weary and wants to keep quiet. *Aggravation from any motion,* even a full inspiration. Cannot endure mental or physical disturbance. *Cannot sit up;* movement from one side of bed to the other is not so bad. Nervous. Lowness of spirits; apprehensive; morose; obstinate; irritable; wishes to be alone. Noise disturbs her. Desires to take a deep, long breath, but cannot easily, as there is a feeling as if the lungs will not expand sufficiently. Nausea or vomiting excited by motion. Burning or pricking or stitching pains. Desire for large quantities of water. Chilliness, with thirst. Head confused, and aching, and heavy. Face hot, red. Mouth and lips dry, with or without thirst. Oppression in the region of the heart. Every spot in the body is painful to pressure. Adapted to brunettes, dark hair, skin and eyes, with firm, fleshy fibre.

CACTUS GRANDIFLORUS.

Labor:

Spasmodic contraction of the os in women who suffer heart spasm (of the circular fibres) and dysmenorrhœa. Painful constriction around the pelvis, extending gradually towards the stomach. Sensation of fulness in the chest.

ABORTION.—

HÆMORRHAGE.—

RETAINED PLACENTA.—

GENERALITIES.—Unwilling to speak a word, or to answer. Knows not why she cries; consolation aggravates. Great sadness. Face blue; cold sweat; pale; flushed. Constriction of various parts. Oppression of the chest, as from a great weight, difficult breathing. Sense as if an iron band prevented normal motion of the chest. *Heart:* constriction as of an iron hand; prickling pain; oppression; dull, heavy pain; pain in apex, shooting down the left arm ; palpitation with vertigo. Whole body feels as if caged, each wire being twisted tighter and tighter. Sensation as though a swarm of hornets were going from the pectoral region to the head.

CALCAREA CARBONICA.

Labor :

Look to the history of the woman. Exhaustion in leuco-phlegmatic women ; much perspiration about the head and the upper part of the body ; every exertion is fatiguing ; cold, clammy, damp feet. Aching in the thighs. Stinging in the os or cervix, stitches. Jerk-like tearing down the sides of the abdomen. Griping and cutting in the hypogastrium. Dragging in the groin. Burning, sore pains in the genitals. Ascending causes vertigo. The least cold air is almost unendurable.

ABORTION.—In leuco-phlegmatic women. Pain in small of back. Colicky or labor-like pain in the uterine region. Pain in the loins. From anæmia ; from leucorrhœa. Disposition to hæmorrhage. Varices of the sexual organs. Usually too profuse and too frequent menses. Cold and damp feet. Vertigo. The history of the case is the principal guide.

HÆMORRHAGE.—Look to the history of the case. In leuco-phlegmatic or plethoric women with light hair, with too profuse, long, and frequent menstruation. Cold, damp feet. Painless hæmorrhage; profuse; worse from motion; bright red blood; caused by least excitement. The saucer-bottom swelling in the pit of the stomach. Vertigo on stooping; worse on rising up again or going upstairs.

GENERALITIES.—The real leuco-phlegmatic constitution. Feels as if she will go crazy. Melancholy. Desire to weep. Fearful apprehensions. Laxness of muscles. Face pale, bloated, blue rings under the eyes. Frequent need to breathe deeply. Twitching of the muscles. Weariness. Sweats easily. Sweat most profuse on head and chest and the upper part of the body. Great heaviness of the body. Congestion to the head. Averse to open air. Chilliness, with desire for warmth and covering.

CAMPHORA.

Labor:
The pains are weak, or cease, and the skin

becomes cold, dry, and shrunken. She does not like to be covered; restlessness. Marble-like coldness of the whole body; very weak pulse. Fainting. (Use the higher potencies.)

ABORTION. — During epidemic influenza. Disposition to catarrhs. Pale, loose, cold skin, with general disposition to catarrhal discharges.

THE BABY.—Where *Antimony tart.* fails, for the same symptoms. Hard places in the skin on the abdomen and thighs, quickly increasing and getting harder; sometimes with a deep redness spreading nearly over the whole abdomen and thighs; violent fever, with startings and tetanic spasms, with bending backwards.

GENERALITIES.— Coldness of the surface of the body to the touch, and in spite of the coldness, the patient throws off all covering, and *will not remain covered.* The face presents a bluish and pinched appearance. *Anxiety.* Face pale. Sensation in eyes as if objects were too bright and shining; pupils contracted. Cramps in the calves. Mucus in the air-passages. Sinking of the vital force, with paleness. *Great weakness.* Mental excitability. Thinking about an existing pain causes it to disappear. Feels very light. Vanishing of all the senses, even touch. Stupor. Fainting. Trembling palpitation, with anxiety. Cramps, with inability to remain covered.

CANNABIS SATIVA.

ABORTION.—In cases where women have been or still are affected with violent gonorrhœa. Also from too frequent sexual intercourse.

GENERALITIES.—Low spirited in the forenoon, cheerful in the afternoon. Urinary complaints; retention; pain during or just after the flow; burning at the beginning and ending of flow. Sensation of hot water being poured over her. Sensation as though cold water were dropping over the heart; over the head; from the anus; or in single parts. Sense of fatigue; of warmth. Dyspnœa.

CANTHARIS.

Labor.—Consult Generalities.

ABORTION.—Constant (at times ineffectual) *desire to urinate*, only a few drops passes at a time, with cutting, burning pain. Pain predominates. From congestion and ulceration of the uterus. Dark flow.

HÆMORRHAGE.—With great irritation of the neck of the bladder. Almost constant desire to urinate, passing only a few drops, with cutting, burning pains during the effort.

RETAINED PLACENTA.—With a teasing to urinate; burning and almost constant desire to urinate. Burning pain in the pelvic portion of the abdomen and in the back; abdomen sensitive; feverishness; vomiting; great anguish and distress; swelling of the lips of the os uteri. Convulsions.

CONVULSIONS.—With dysuria and hydrophobic symptoms. Bright light on objects, and the sight, sound, or drinking of water, or the mere touch, seem to reproduce the spasms, which are usually violent. Renewal of spasms from touching the larynx or painful parts. Face swollen and puffy. Urine scalding, dark, and scanty, with frequent desire. Albuminuria, cylindrical casts, mucus, and shreds in urine. Vulva swollen and sensitive. With retained placenta or membranes, eyes bright, pupils dilated widely. Face pale and yellowish, bearing an expression of deep-seated suffering.

GENERALITIES. — Moaning. Lamenting. Restlessness. Face pale; wretched; sickly appearance. Urine scanty; painful; flaky; like pus; reddish. Teasing to urinate, worse standing, still more so walking. Violent cutting and burning pain in bladder before, during, and after urination. Expels moles, dead fœtus and placenta when indicated. Worse from drinking cold water; while urinating; after urinating. Irritable. Whining and complaining. Paroxysms of rage, with crying, barking, and beating; renewed by the sight of dazzling, bright objects; when touching the larynx, or when trying to drink water. Death-like look during and after pains. Thirst, with aversion to all fluids. Anxiety about the heart; palpitation. Weakness. Prostration. Faintness. Raw and sore pain in the whole body; every part sensitive.

CARBO VEGETABILIS.
Labor :

The pains are too weak, or cease from great debility. Varicose condition of the vulva. After great loss of animal fluids, or other debilitating effects of previous or existing disease. *Fainting* from weakness, caused by loss of animal fluids; after sleeping. Much belching of wind, or eructations.

ABORTION.—Menses have been too pale or scanty, or too copious and premature, with a decided varicose condition of the sexual organs; frequent headache; abdominal spasms.

HÆMORRHAGE.—Passive. Continuous. She is already cold, skin bluish or deathly pale; pulse rapid and weak. Excessive prostration. Burning pain across the sacrum and lower part of the spine, with burning pains in the chest and difficult breathing. Patient wants to be fanned. Much itching of the vulva and anus. Dragging pains from abdomen to back. Hardly any restlessness; no anxiety. Blood pale or thick, or of various appearance.

CONVULSIONS.—Collapse and heart failure; labor-pains weak and ceasing, with great debility; breath cold and short, with cold hands and feet; desire to be fanned, must have more air.

AFTER-PAINS. — *Pains turn up in distant parts from the pelvic region*, with exacerbations and remissions occurring as regularly as if they were in the uterus.

GENERALITIES.—Stupor; collapse. Wants to be fanned, wants the windows opened. must have more air. Head hot. Anguish. Irritable. Obstructed flatulency. Respiration oppressed. Pulse imperceptible; small; soft; thready. Biting, pungent, or burning pains on external parts of the body. Sense of a plug in the back. Better from eructations. Confusion of head. Indifference. Headache as from constriction of the scalp. Face hippocratic; very pale; greenish; pointed nose; cold sweat; cold; cheeks red and covered with cold sweat. Vital force nearly exhausted; lies as if dead; breath cool. Faint-like weakness.

CAULOPHYLLUM.

Labor:

Extremely rigid os uteri; pains like pricking of needles in cervix. *Severe, spasmodic,* intermittent, short, irregular pains, *without progress.* Pains flag from exhaustion, on account of the long continuance of the labor; too weak to develop normal pains. Thirsty and feverish. Spasmodic, inefficient pains in various parts of the abdomen. Great exhaustion. Severe contractions of the fundus and constriction of the os uteri ; spasmodic contraction of the os. Drawing in the uterine ligaments. Spasmodic pains, flying from one place to another, but *not* going in the normal or right direction. Nausea and spasmodic pains in the stomach. Profuse secretion of mucus from the vagina. Tormenting, useless pains in the beginning of labor.

Nearest the specific for *false pains*. Stops the false and develops genuine pains.

ABORTION.—Severe pain in the back and loins, with great want of uterine tonicity. Feeble uterine contractions, tormenting, irregular, and attended with *very slight hæmorrhage*. Pain predominating. Passive discharge. Spasmodic bearing down. Vascular excitement. From uterine congestion, passive ; from hysteria ; from uterine inertia ; from rheumatism.

HÆMORRHAGE.—Uterine debility. *Profuse* hæmorrhage from a relaxed or feebly contracting uterus *after hasty labor*. Passive oozing. Tremulous weakness felt over the entire body, accompanying the flow, with sense of exhaustion. Uterus is soft and relaxed, and contracts very feebly. Especially after natural or hasty labor.

RETAINED PLACENTA.—Spasmodic retention; from exhaustion and weakness; no contractions; flooding.

CONVULSIONS.—Spasms during labor, with very moist genitals and spasmodically contracted os. With very weak and irregular pains. She feels very weak, and is feverish and thirsty.

AFTER-PAINS.—Spasmodic pains in the lower abdomen (or in other parts), sometimes extending into the groins. *Particularly after protracted and exhausting labor*. Pains in the back and chest. She is nervous, sleepless, weak.

GENERALITIES.—According to Farrington the main characteristic is intermittency of pains. They are usually sharp and crampy, and appear in bladder, groins, and lower extremities. Extreme uterine atony. In nervous women in whom pain seems to be insupportable. Exhaustion of the whole system. She can scarcely speak at times, so weak is the voice. False labor-pains during the last weeks of pregnancy, consisting of painful bearing-down sensations in the hypogastrium. Patient is fretful and easily displeased. Headache, with pressure behind the eyes. Neuralgia of the vagina, when the vagina is excessively irritable and the pain and spasms are intense and continued. Hysteria and uterine displacements. Rheumatism, especially of the *small joints*. Painful stiffness of the affected joints. A sort of vertigo, with dimness of sight. Moth spots on the forehead, with leucorrhœa. Thirst.

CAUSTICUM.

Labor :

After debility, night-watching, grief, or some depressing influence. Distressing, sore aching pain in her back is the chief complaint, with spasmodic labor-pains. *Uterine inertia, with great relaxation of the tissues* and prostration. Paralytic condition of fundus of the bladder, with inability to urinate. Numb feeling. Labor-pains insufficient, irregular ; os dilated, but the woman has become tired and fretful.

CONVULSIONS.—With screams, gnashing of the teeth, and violent movement of the limbs. Dyspnœa, with frequent sighing. Jerkings, with feverish heat and coldness of hands and feet.

GENERALITIES.—In scrofulous women, or those having a weakened or emaciated appearance. This weakness may result from grief of long standing, or from some diseased condition. The skin often has a dirty-white look. Sadness. Whining mood. Very suspicious and mistrustful. Noises in the ears in general; a constant roaring before the ears; humming or tinkling in ears; reverberation of all sounds in the ears. Upper eyelids drop. Sudden and frequent loss of sight, with sensation of a film before the eyes. In cough is obliged to swallow what is raised. Burning, in itching blotches, like nettle-rash. Motion rendered difficult, muscles being shortened. Full of timorous fancies. Retention of urine, with frequent and urging desire; dribbling of but a few drops. Shortness of breath. Stitches about the heart. Stitches in the back; in left lumbar region. Bruised pain in the coccyx. Weakness and trembling. Faint-like sinking of strength. Restlessness of the body. Yawning and stretching.

CHAMOMILLA.

Labor:

Distressing spasmodic pains. Very sensitive to the pains; she can hardly bear them; she wishes to get away from herself and from the pains; almost frantic; great impatience. She is very fretful, cross, unreasonable, and peevish, cannot bear any one near her; cannot return a civil answer. She is very spiteful or cries out sharply. Hour-glass contractions; thirst; desire for fresh air; restlessness; more or less discharge of dark coagulated blood from the vagina. Pains ceasing. Pains too weak. Fainting from sensitiveness to the pains, with vertigo, dimness of vision, dullness of hearing, and nausea; must have fresh air and fresh water. False labor-pains—abdominal pains with *frequent emissions of large quantities of pale urine.* Pains force the child upward. *Tearing pains beginning in the back* and radiating down the inner side of the legs. Passes quantities of colorless urine with the pains. Says she must and will get up. One cheek red, the other pale. Rigid os uteri. Great nervous excitement; the labor is extremely painful; she moans, laments, and calls for

5

assistance. Drawing from the sacral region forward, griping and pinching in the uterus, followed by large clots of blood (Placenta prævia ?). Snappish in the first stage, and will not permit an examination; sends the doctor away and sends for him soon again. Has a very poor opinion of her attendant, and tells him so plainly. Not satisfied with anything he may do for her.

ABORTION.—Threatened from anger. Pains predominate. Spiteful, snappish irritability, unreasonable. Pains and dark clotted blood with *frequent profuse urination;* passes colorless urine with every pain; colicky pains in the uterine region. Discharge dark or black; offensive; coagulated; in bright-red gushes; profuse. Contracting, out-pressing pains from back to front, worse lying in bed. *Labor-like pains in the uterine region* alternating with hæmorrhage; extending into hypochondrium; into thighs; periodical. Pain, restlessness, and agony referred to the uterine region. Nervous excitement. Heaviness of abdomen. Yawning, chills, and shuddering.

HÆMORRHAGE.—Dark coagulated blood, occasionally interrupted by bright-red gushes, with tearing pains in the legs and violent labor-pains in the uterus. Of dark blood, with pressure toward the uterus and frequent discharge of colorless urine. Flowing by fits and starts of irregular intervals. *From anger.* Frequent pressure toward uterus like labor-pains. Sensation as if the sacrum were being separated. Through abdominal walls the uterus can be felt to be contracted into little knots about the size of a walnut. Discharge dark; profuse; dark clots or coagulated; black; fœtid; putrid; lumpy; intermittent; convulsive; with frequent discharge of colorless urine. During or after labor.

RETAINED PLACENTA.—Hour-glass contractions with the general indications of the remedy. See under *Labor.*

CONVULSIONS. Powerful. *From a fit of anger.* Excessive sensitiveness of the rigid os. Labor-pains spasmodic and distressing, tearing down the limbs. Irritability and petulance; spiteful excitability. One cheek red, the other pale. Starts and shocks during sleep. Convulsions in the back, with throwing backward of the head, and stiffness of the body, as in tetanus, or of a tetanic nature.

AFTER-PAINS.—Violent and distressing,

rendering her frantic and ill-natured, spiteful. Lochia profuse and dark, clotted. Wants fresh air. Feels that she cannot endure the pains; she wants to get away from herself. Thirst. One of the best remedies when indicated.

GENERALITIES.—*A spiteful, sudden, or uncivil irritability.* She feels as if she "can't be civil," "cannot give a civil answer," is very snappish and sharp or short in speaking. Suffering from fits of anger. Calmness contra-indicates this remedy. Very irritable. Severity of the pains makes her cross; too severe to be borne. Abdominal pains, with frequent emissions of pale, colorless urine in large quantities. Desire to lie down; to be in motion. Yawning and stretching of the limbs. Thirst. Chilliness with thirst. Cheeks very red; one cheek red, the other pale. Sensation of anxiousness in the body (restlessness). Cannot endure being spoken to, or interrupted while speaking. Great impatience, everything seems to go too slowly. Peevish, nothing pleases. Touchy from the slightest disturbance or contradiction. Sensitive to all odors. Breathing oppressed as if chest were not wide enough. Palpitation and faintness. Drawing pains in the back; small of back feels bruised. Sensation as if the lumbar region would be broken, with dragging and drawing pains extending from the region of the liver, over the abdomen and deep into the pelvis, when lying in bed. Bad results of Morphine or Opium.

CHINA OFFICINALIS.

Labor :

Pains cease from hæmorrhage, a protracted diarrhœa, etc, Atony of the uterus. She cannot bear to be touched (even the hands) during a pain. Digging, tearing pains in the uterus. Fainting and convulsions from the loss of blood and other animal fluids. Desire to be fanned gently. Desire to have fresh air. *Ringing in the ears, cold skin, loss of pulse* (or nearly so), *and cold sweat.* Vertigo. Exhaustion from loss of fluids. Intolerance of examination from nervousness.

ABORTION.—Sensation of distension, or as if bloated, of the abdomen, as if it were packed full. She wishes to discharge flatus, but its passage upward or downward, gives

no relief. Hæmorrhage and its sequelæ.
The membranes of an early ovum remain
for weeks, keeping up a constant hæmorrhage. Profuse bright-red hæmorrhage, with
most alarming prostration. She may be
unconscious, pulseless, breathless, limp and pallid.
Hæmorrhage predominates. From anæmia ;
uterine congestion ; uterine inertia. Discharge black and clotted ; dark ; in bright-
red gushes ; intermittent ; passive ; profuse ;
watery, with clots.

HÆMORRHAGE.—From atony of the uterus.
From abuse of Chamomile. Paroxysmal
discharge of clots of dark blood. Uterine
spasms, colic. Frequent urging to urinate,
and painful tension in the abdomen. Coldness and blueness of the skin. Suitable to
persons who have lost much blood, even in
severe cases, with heaviness of the head ;
ringing in the ears ; vertigo ; vanishing of
the senses ; sopor ; fainting fits ; cold extremities ; gasping for breath ; pale and
bluish face and hands ; with convulsive
jerks across the abdomen ; twitching and
jerking of single muscles. Intermitting
with uterine cramps, colic and painful distension of the abdomen. She sees persons

or objects on closing the eyes; these disappear as soon as the eyes are opened. Wants to be fanned gently. Fainting. Discharge black; dark clots; clots mixed with pale watery blood; very profuse; passive.

RETAINED PLACENTA.—Attended by hæmorrhage, as above.

CONVULSIONS.—*From great loss of blood.* Rush of blood to the head, throbbing carotids. Twitching of the limbs.

THE BABY.—Syncope, after great loss of blood by the mother during labor.

GENERALITIES.—Swarthy skin. Debility of the system from the loss of fluids, whether much or little. Sensitive in the whole nervous system; the least noise or excitement is unendurable. Ringing in the ears. Face pale; red; red spots on cheeks; blue color around the eyes; sallow complexion; hollow eyes. Hunger without appetite. Chilliness, with shivering. Great thirst. Pain as if bruised in various parts. Tearing, jerking, craping, sensations. Congestion of single parts. Fainting from loss of animal fluids. Lassitude of the body; wants to sit down or rest. Desire for motion. Nervous debility; general debility.

Shuddering of single parts. Slow train of ideas. Delirium after depletion. Inclined to reproach and vex others. She thinks she is very unfortunate and constantly harrassed by enemies. Low-spirited, gloomy, has no desire to live. Inconsolable anxiety, even to suicide. Enlarged spleen. Palpitation with rush of blood to the face. Heat of the face, with cold body. Single parts feel pithy, numb. Intolerance of sensual impressions. Intense throbbing headache. *Slight touch* aggravates the pain, which is relieved by a *firm, steady pressure*. In breathing a *puffing* noise is produced. She can only distinguish the outlines of distant objects. When reading, the letters appear pale and surrounded by a white border. She sees better after sleeping. Sensation in abdomen of distension.

CHININUM SULFURICUM.

Labor:

Labor-pains appear like tonic spasms, accompanied by convulsive twitchings. Unconsciousness after parturition. Oppressed respiration. Distended veins of the head and neck; rapid and intermitting pulse;

albuminuria. During intervals convulsive action of muscles of face, eyes, etc.

HÆMORRHAGE.—Passive metrorrhagia, with diminished irritability. Great debility from considerable loss of blood.

CONVULSIONS.—Tetanic convulsions, with loss of consciousness; during intervals convulsive action of muscles of face, eyes, etc. Oppressed respiration. Distended veins in head and neck; weak, rapid, intermitting pulse and albuminuria. Unconsciousness after labor. Albuminuric spasms. Twitching or clonic spasms in limbs.

GENERALITIES.—Buoyancy, excited state; later despondency. Feeling of impending evil; anxiety. Whirling in head like a mill-wheel. Violent throbbing headache. Closes eyelids involuntarily from sheer prostration. Can see objects only when looking sideways. Ringing, roaring, buzzing in the ears. Face pale; suffering; sickly; puffy. Restlessness; excessive sensibility to touch and noises. Weakness. Trembling. Nervousness. Faintness. Hunger. Debility caused by considerable loss of fluids. Enlarged spleen; dull pains in, disappear on pressure. Enlarged and congested liver.

CHLOROFORM.

Labor:

No freedom from suffering between the pains.
She complains much of her back or of extreme pain and tenderness over the whole abdomen. Very restless. Cannot find rest in any position, tosses about and is very restless. Protracted and severe labor from rigidity of the os uteri. Women subject to convulsions during labor. Complete paralysis of sphincter vesicæ after labor.

CONVULSIONS.—Women subject to convulsions during labor. From anæmia; uræmia; reflex irritation.

CICUTA VIROSA.

Labor:

CONVULSIONS.—Strange contortions of upper part of body and limbs during the paroxysms, with blue face and *frequent interruptions of breathing for a few moments,* followed by weakness, and insensibility, as if dead. Cold, pale face. Half-closed eyes with blue margins. Opisthotonos, jerks as from electric shocks, from the head through the body. Borborygmus. Hiccough and belching. *Convulsions, especially after delivery, of excessive violence.* Rigid, with fixed staring eyes. Frothing at the mouth. Jaws locked. Bites the tongue.

THE BABY.—Spasmodic rigidity. Child seems well and in good spirits, when suddenly it becomes rigid, followed by relaxation and great prostration.

GENERALITIES.—Excessive moaning and howling. She does rash and absurd things. Is very violent in all her actions. Repeated movements of the head, as twitching, jerking, throwing the head back, etc. Contraction of the pupils of the eyes. The letters seem to move about when she is reading. Violent jerks of the muscles; motion is convulsive. Worse from turning the head. Feels as if in a strange place, causes fear. Answers short. Face deathly pale and cold; red; bluish; puffed up. Distortions of the face, either horrible or ridiculous. Grinding of the teeth. Foam in and about the mouth. Inability to swallow. Sudden shocks deep in the pit of the stomach causes opisthotonos. Feels as if the heart stopped beating. Frequent involuntary jerking and twitching in arms and fingers. Trembling of left leg. Tonic spasm renewed from the slightest

touch; from opening the door; from loud
talking. Sensation in many parts as from a
bruise.

CIMICIFUGA RACEMOSA.

Labor:

False labor-pains, spasmodic, neuralgic,
rheumatic, in uterus, a few days or even
weeks before labor sets in. Pains under left
breast changing to left ovary or arm. *Rigors
or nervous chills (shivering) in the first stage of
labor.* Spasmodic rigidity of the os, causing
pains to be ineffectual. Continuous tearing,
distressing pains, during which the uterus
seems to ascend. Pains fly from side to side
in abdomen (Ip., Lyc.) and double her up.
Nervous excitement in rheumatic women.
Labor-pains severe, tedious; spasmodic with
fainting fits or cramps, *but are not located
properly to effect expulsion;* worse from least
noise. Limbs heavy and torpid. Uterine
rheumatism. Entire cessation of labor-pains.
Pains cease from hæmorrhage Irregularly
constricted os; at one time dilated and dilatable, then suddenly closed by spasm. Melancholy and nervous; irritating choreic motions all over. Headache, with impairment

of vision. Crying out in agony. Declares
she will go crazy, and her actions indicate
the danger. Suspicious. Her talk is nonsensical, and yet she seems to be conscious
of what she is doing, and says she cannot
help it. Visions of rats, etc. Cramps in the
hips during labor, crying out and complaining about her hips. Cardiac neuralgia. Despondency. She is of a rheumatic diathesis;
subject to rheumatic pains.

ABORTION.—Habitual, in women of rheumatic tendencies. Cold chills and pricking
sensations in mammæ. *Pains fly across abdomen from side to side*, especially from right
to left, and seem to double her up, Subinvolution. Convulsions with labor-pains.
From or following fright. Pains predominate. Pain in back, extending into thighs.
Labor-like pains in uterine region. From
uterine congestion; uterine inertia; rheumatism. At the third month.

HÆMORRHAGE.—Discharge profuse, dark,
and coagulated, more of a passive character,
accompanied with heavy, pressing-down,
labor-like pains, nervous, hysteric spasms,
pain in the back and limbs simulating rheumatism. Pains cease from hæmorrhage.

RETAINED PLACENTA.—Rheumatic subjects. There is a distressing, tearing pain in the uterine region. No uterine action. Feels sore; headache; brain feels too large for the skull; eyeballs pain.

CONVULSIONS. — False labor-pains, sharp pains across abdomen, insomnia. Labor-pains severe, tedious, spasmodic, with fainting fits or cramps. Cardiac neuralgia during parturition. From nervous excitement. Feels strange, talks incoherently, screams, tries to injure herself. Shivers during first stage of labor. Preceded by great mental excitement, with visions of objects not present, and are followed by languor, and relaxation of the whole system. The paroxysms are very violent. *With spasmodically contracted or rigid os.*

AFTER-PAINS.—*Worse in the groins.* Oversensitiveness; nausea and vomiting. Great tenderness on pressure, womb does not contract properly. Pains cause flushing of the face, and in right side of head, back of orbits. She is low-spirited, restless, sleepless, predisposed to neuralgia, very sensitive to impressions, and feels her pains very acutely; cannot tolerate the pains.

GENERALITIES.—During labor she has a horribly apprehensive mood. She has a dread or fear of something about to happen. In all her mental symptoms there is a want of natural coherence. Thinks she is going crazy, and imagines all sorts of strange appearances, and that some one is going to kill her. Incessant talk in which she is constantly changing from one subject to another. She is despondent and seems to feel under a heavy black cloud. Feels that the top of her head would fly off. Pain as if a bolt had been driven from the neck to the vertex, worse at every throb of the heart. Headache down to the nose. Pain in eyeballs or temples; shooting into eyeballs, very severe. Sensible to the least noise, with the spasmodic pains. Every inhalation seems to bring the cold air into contact with the brain. Face bluish; wild, fearful expression. Forehead cold; deadly pale. Suddenly very faint, face ashy white. Excessive muscular soreness; general bruised feeling as if sore. Fear of death; thinks she is going to die. Fainting fits. Spasms of the broad ligaments. Cough at every attempt to speak. Pain in the region of the heart,

all over the chest and down the left arm;
palpitation. Dyspnœa. Heart's action
ceases suddenly; impending suffocation.
Pulse weak, irregular. Aching in the limbs.
Uneasy feeling in the limbs, causing restlessness. Trembling of the legs, twitching of
the flexors; legs unsteady. Cramps in the
extremities, and even intermitting spasms.
Hysterical spasms. Pains come on suddenly.
Pricking all over. Like electric shocks here
and there. Numbness.

CINNAMOMUM.

Labor:

Weak, ineffectual, or false labor-pains.
Spasms, twitchings, or fainting during labor.
Complete cessation of labor-pains. *Severe
flooding in primipara after first few pains,* when
the os has dilated about an inch; *placenta
descends with the head.*

ABORTION.—Profuse flow of *bright-red blood
after a strain* in the loins; from a false step;
from over exertion. Hæmorrhage predominates.

HÆMORRHAGE. — *Bright-red flow* from a
strain, misstep, or some exertion. Profuse.
Sudden. *Severe flooding in primipara after*

first few pains. Soon, or some days after delivery metrorrhagia, unaccompanied by plethora. Profuse; passive; with or without pain. From chlorosis or anæmia.

CONVULSIONS.—Spasms, or twitchings, or fainting during labor.

AFTER-PAINS.—Mitigates after-pains.

GENERALITIES.—In the lymphatic, feeble and cachectic. With a lax tissue and languid circulation, a great tendency to hysteria, and always worse by any lifting or exertion.

COCCULUS INDICUS.

Labor:

Spasmodic, irregular, *paralytic pains.* Pains weak; ceasing. One hard pain, and then after a longer interval several lighter ones. Much headache. Numb, paralyzed feeling in the lower limbs, with trembling. Paralyzed weakness, worse in hips and lower limbs. Spasmodic pains in the uterus, with nausea and vomiting. Fainting. Terrible pain in the small of the back, with hour-glass contractions. Mental terror during spasmodic, irregular pains. Weak and nervous women.

ABORTION.—Much bilious vomiting. Paralytic pain in the back, rendering the lower extremities nearly useless.

HÆMORRHAGE.—Scanty.

RETAINED PLACENTA.—Hour-glass contraction. Terrible pains in the small of the back; lower limbs feel paralyzed; frequent vomiting.

CONVULSIONS.—Spasms following difficult labor, and then brought on by changing the woman's position, passing off with a sigh. *Exalted susceptibility to impressions*, everything causes starting and trembling all over the body. Shuddering. Mental terror during spasmodic, irregular pains. Rapid oscillation of the eyeballs beneath the closed lids. Weak and nervous women. Irritable weakness. From prolonged loss of sleep.

GENERALITIES.—Sensation as of sharp stones in the abdomen at every movement. Painful pressure in the uterus, with cramps in the chest and fainting nausea. Debilitated as to the cerebro-spinal nervous system. Weak, nervous temperament; light-haired females, especially those suffering from uterine complaints or menstrual difficulties, or troubles during pregnancy. *Sensations* of hollowness; as if bruised in outer parts or in bones; numb feeling; pricking, knocking, or throbbing in inner parts; pain as if paralyzed; pressing together, as if single parts had gone to sleep. Laxness of muscles. Spasms in inner parts. Spasms, which occur frequently at midnight. Shuddering in general. Shivering over the mammæ. Paleness of the skin; red spots. Stupid feeling in the head. Thoughts fixed on one unpleasant subject; she is absorbed and observes nothing about her. Sobbing, moaning, and groaning. Sudden great anxiety. Starts very easily. Very easily offended; every trifle makes her angry. Face pale; blue around the eyes. Cold sweat on face. Menses during pregnancy. Sense of constriction of the throat, causing obstructed breathing. Cracking in the knee-joints (and others) when moving. Involuntary motions of right arm and right leg, ceases during sleep. Feels too weak to talk loud. Anæmic states. Her head feels worse after eating or drinking. Headache, as if the eyes would be torn out, particularly on motion, with vertigo.

COFFEA CRUDUM.

Labor :

Ineffectual labor-pains; contractions of uterus and pressure upon os uteri, causing only pain in small of back. She feels every pain intensely, weeps and laments with constant and extreme fear of death. Pains, though severe, are not efficacious. Pains insupportable to her feelings. False labor-pains very distressing in abdomen, and facial neuralgia. Feels as if she will "go distracted." Nervous excitement. Labor-pains ceasing, with complaining loquacity. Rigidity of vulva and perinæum, with nervous sensitiveness. Fainting in highly sensitive persons after a fright (if *Acon.* fails).

ABORTION.—Excessively severe pains from threatened abortion. From general excitation.

HÆMORRHAGE.—*Passes large black lumps*, worse from every motion, with violent pains in the groin and fear of death with despair. With excessive sensitiveness of the organs and voluptuous itching; she would like to scratch, but there is too great sensibility.

CONVULSIONS.—*From extreme excitability* of the nervous system when spasms are apprehended. Head hot, red. Face puffed, eyes glistening; after sudden emotions, especially pleasing ones. Constant loquacity and sleeplessness. Cold extremities. Grinding of the teeth.

AFTER-PAINS.—Painfulness out of proportion to the contractions of the uterus. Distressed: she cannot bear them; extreme fear of death. She is sleepless, or she is very sleepy but cannot sleep.

GENERALITIES.—Ecstatic state of mind; gayety. Over-excited state of the mind: Fear of death is usually present with severe pain. Cannot bear even a slight pain, which causes great complaint and crying and whining. The senses are all too acute. Distant noises seem to be magnified. Mental or bodily irritability. Nervous excitement. Acute hearing. *Tight* pain; rending pain. *Sleeplessness.* Sleepless after labor. Drowsiness, but cannot sleep. Excessive weeping and lamentations over trifles. Bad effects from sudden pleasurable surprises. Violent, irregular palpitation of the heart, with trembling of limbs. Twitching of the limbs. Physical excitement through mental exaltation. Fainting from sudden emotions.

Headache, with *intense* pain, the head feeling *contracted* or as if *too small*.

CONIUM MACULATUM.

Labor:

Pains spasmodic. Spasmodic contractions of the os uteri, with stinging, stitching pains. Vertigo, particularly on turning in bed. Scirrhosis in the mammæ or uterus. Very sensitive across the abdomen. Complete sleeplessness and exhaustion during parturition. Extreme sensitiveness to light. Hourglass contractions.

ABORTION.—From shocks; from falls; from concussions. Vertigo on turning over when lying down. The flow of urine intermits. Induration of cervix.

RETAINED PLACENTA.—Hour-glass contractions. See under *Labor*.

AFTER-PAINS.—By putting babe to breast, pains extending from left to right.

GENERALITIES.—Great dizziness brought on when lying down, and when moving the head ever so slightly, or even the eyes—all contents of the room appearing to whirl around. She wishes to keep the head *perfectly still*. Urine flows in a full stream, then stops, flows again, stops, etc. Old contusions and sprains. Pains in the glands, as from contusions. Wasting away of glands; itching of; induration of; sensibility of; hard swelling of; tingling in. When the mammæ have been injured recently or for a long time. Heartburn. Sensation of a hoop, band, or something tight around parts. Face bluish; reddish-yellow. Hysterics. Yellow nails. Indifference. Morose. Ringing, humming, roaring in the ears. Picking of the nose till it bleeds; finger tips. Terrible nausea and vomiting during pregnancy. Stitches as from needles in left mamma. Cracking of knee-joints. Trembling in all the limbs.

CROCUS SATIVUS.

Labor :

ABORTION.—Sensation as if something alive moved in the abdomen, with nausea, faintness, and hæmorrhage, aggravated or caused by the least movement. *Black, stringy blood* with little clots adhering. Hæmorrhage predominates. At the third month. At the first month from overheating. Discharge *black ; stringy ;* coagulated ; offensive ;

dark; passive; profuse; *worse from motion;* partly bright, partly composed of black strings; as fast as the blood flows from vulva it forms clots or stringy masses.

HÆMORRHAGE.—Sensation of rolling or bounding in the abdomen, as of something alive. Great exhaustion. Cutting pain deep in lower abdomen, extending to back. Icy-cold feet. Fainting. Great excitement. Palpitations. Violent cephalic throbbings. *Dark, stringy* blood hanging down from the bleeding os. From a false step; lifting; strain in the loins; after least motion; from overheating. Discharge active; passive; *worse from motion;* black clotted; *dark; stringy; viscid;* fœtid; offensive.

RETAINED PLACENTA.—Shortly after delivery placenta still retained, hæmorrhage in large clots; womb dilated, soft; fainting, pulseless, extremities icy-cold; anxious palpitations, with a desire to draw a long breath.

GENERALITIES.—Hysteria with choreic symptoms. This remedy causes jumping, dancing, laughing, whistling, desire to kiss other people. Angry, and then suddenly repents. Alternation of anger, talking, laughing. Sensation of something moving in the abdomen or in the pit of the stomach. Abdomen swollen. Sense of fatigue. Mist before the eyes. Yawning. Drowsiness. Sings involuntarily when hearing others sing. Restless, anxious, sorrowful mood. Must wink and wipe eyes frequently, as though a film of mucus was over them. The light seems dimmer than usual. Feeling in eyes as after much weeping. Inclined to press eyelids together tightly. Jerking in muscles. Sings in sleep.

CROTALUS HORRIDUS.

ABORTION.—During the course of a septic or zymotic disease, or from other blood-poisoning (*Pyrogen*). Blood dark, fluid, offensive.

HÆMORRHAGE.—Dizziness, confusion, or deep coma. Broken-down constitutions. Blood dark, fluid, offensive.

CONVULSIONS.—In connection with albuminuria, torpor, coma. Bloated countenance. Sensation as of tight constriction in throat. Tremulous weakness all over, as if some evil were apprehended. Hysterical convulsions, followed by paralysis. Septic or zymotic influence (*Pyrogen*), or in hæmorrhage or broken-down constitutions. Trembling of the limbs. Foaming at mouth. Violent cries, delirium.

GENERALITIES.—Nervous agitation. Sensitive. Irritable, cross, snappish. Mental delusions. Delirium, with wide open eyes. Restless. Broken-down constitutions. Sadness. Weeping. Fainting on sitting up. Oozing of blood from any part. Great thirst. Breathing embarrassed. Palpitation as if heart tumbled about. Tremulous weakness, as from impending evil. Torpor, drowsiness, coma. Yellow skin. Affects the nerves and blood.

CUPRUM METALLICUM.
Labor :

Great restlessness between the pains. Violent spasmodic pains at irregular intervals, often with cramping in the lower limbs; or cramps in the fingers and toes only. Hour-glass contractions with distressing cramps in the uterus, and the hands and feet. (Cupr. Ars.).

RETAINED PLACENTA.—Hour-glass contractions, as above.

CONVULSIONS.—*With or preceded by violent vomiting*. Opisthotonos with every spasm, with spreading out of the limbs and opening of the mouth. Spasms begin as cramps in the fingers and toes, or in the whole extremities; or even in the abdomen. Clonic spasms *during* pregnancy, when the attacks begin at the periphery and spread centrally. Post-partum, with rash. Sour-smelling sweat. Soreness of abdomen to pressure. Burning in small of back. Shrill, piercing shrieks before fits. Frequent attacks of blind rage, biting at persons (Cupr. Ars.). Fingers clenched. Marked blueness of face and mouth. Any attempt to swallow fluids causes gurgling in the throat. Great restlessness between the attacks.

AFTER-PAINS.—Terrible cramping spasms, often with cramps of the extremities, including the fingers and toes (Cupr. Acet.) Severe headache. Especially in the multiparæ.

GENERALITIES.—*Cupr. Acet.*, and *Cupr. Met.*, are generally conceded to have the same set of symptoms. *Strong metallic* (coppery) *taste in the mouth* (Rhus). Spasmodic affections generally, especially in the fingers, toes, or pit of stomach. Movements of the head. Respiration oppressed; unequal. Face bluish; bluish-red. Severe vomiting. Motions convulsive. Bloated skin. Weeping. Afraid of every one who approaches in delirium. Sadness. Full of fears. Restless tossing about. Tossing about of the head. Eyes dim. Quick rotation of eyeballs with lids closed. Face pale; very red; blue; grayish, dirty; pinched; sunken features; icy-cold. Lips blue. Foam at mouth. Swallow of cold water relieves vomiting. Anxious feeling about the heart. Twitching of the limbs. Cramps of calves. Nervous trembling.

DIGITALIS PURPUREA.

Labor:

Fainting. *Pulse very slow,* thin and irregular, missing the third, fifth or seventh beat. Cold sweat and death-like countenance.

ABORTION.—Distressing nausea and vomiting in the incipiency of abortion, accompanied by deathly faint, sinking sensation at pit of stomach. Surface of body cold, and often accompanied with cold sweat. Flow of blood from vagina.

GENERALITIES.—Dependent on stagnation of blood in consequence of defects of heart. Debility. Emaciation. Extreme thirst. Constant *icy-coldness despite warm covering*. Constant restlessness, fear of death. Great prostration. Sad, depressed, anxious. Breathing deep, sighing, slower than normal. Desire to take a deep breath, but lungs do not seem to expand sufficiently to get more than a half-breath. Cough caused by deep breathing. Suffocative spells with painful constriction of the chest. Pulse either *slow*, or *feeble*, or becoming *irregular*. *A very slow pulse is the chief characteristic*. Bluish appearance of the face; pale; deathlike. Stool gray or ash-colored. Urine scanty. Heart beat intermits the third, fifth or seventh. Fainting. Tearful, low-spirited. Persistent nausea and vomiting. Sensation if she moved that the heart would cease to beat, with fear of impending death.

DULCAMARA.

ABORTION.—When induced by a cold, damp place, as in a milk-house or cellar.

GENERALITIES.—Aggravation from cold, damp weather or from changes from hot to cold weather, especially of sudden changes. Twitching of the muscles of the mouth or eyelids when the weather is damp. Colic from cold, especially with diarrhœa at night. Tongue paralyzed in damp weather, with impaired speech. Bright-red eruptions. Inclined to scold without being angry. Restlessness. Saliva tenacious, soap-like. Convulsions beginning in the face. One-sided spasms; speechless.

ERIGERON CANADENSE.

Labor :

Flooding before and after, with violent irritation of rectum and bladder.

ABORTION.—Hæmorrhage after. Diarrhœa. Dysuria. With prolapse of the uterus.

HÆMORRHAGE.—Very profuse flow of bright-red blood ; alarmingly increased by every movement ; with irritation of the rectum and bladder. Dysuria. Pallor and weakness in consequence of the loss of blood. Comes with a sudden gush and then stops again. May flow-in fits and starts.

May be kept in check to a certain extent by remaining perfectly still.

GENERALITIES.—Painful urination, with or without bloody urine. Congestion of the head, red face, nosebleed; febrile action. Violent retching and burning in the stomach, with vomiting of blood.

FERRUM METALLICUM.

Labor:

Feeling very weak, even from talking. Wishes to lie down, face and lips very pale, or the cheeks may be fiery-red. Frequent attacks of tremor, alternating with a sensation of extreme weakness, as if very weary. Trembling of the whole body. With each pain the face flushes up fiery-red. Spasmodic labor-pains. Dryness of the vagina.

ABORTION.—Pains and flowing accompanied with a fiery-red face. Paleness. Weakness. Atony of the sexual organs. Great tendency to abortion. Excessive nervous erethism and flowing. From anæmia; from inertia; from nervous sensibility. Discharge profuse; dark; coagulated; watery with clots.

HÆMORRHAGE.—With fiery-red face and

hard full pulse. Hæmorrhagic tendency. With pains in loins and labor-like colic in weakly women. Breathing rapid and a little labored. Blood coagulates easily. Chilly with fiery-red face and thirst. Flow bright-red, often mixed with coagula and is associated with a great deal of flushing. Pale watery flow, with pale lips and face. Flow partly fluid and partly black clotted, with violent labor-like pains, full, hard pulse and frequent short shudderings; headache, vertigo, hot urine and great weakness. From the use of Quinine.

AFTER-PAINS.—Feeble women with fiery-red faces. Violent labor-like pains in the loins and abdomen, with discharge of partly fluid and partly clotted blood. Full hard pulse. Frequent short shuddering, headache and vertigo.

GENERALITIES.—Weakness and great debility. Face fiery-red; sallow; reddish yellow; red spots on cheeks; very pale; flushing with the pains. Great variability of the mind. Head confused, muddled. Prone to weep, or to laugh, immoderately. Congestion to the head. Head hot, feet cold. Ringing in the ears. Vagina dry. Palpitation, better walking slowly. Restless, must walk slowly about. So weak she must lie down. Red parts become white. Cracking in the joints. Pseudo-plethora is the key-note. The Ferrum patient is usually a cold patient. The least contradiction angers.

GELSEMIUM SEMPERVIRENS.

Labor:

Rigid Os Uteri. Cutting pains in the abdomen from in front and below, upward and backward, rendering every labor-pain useless. *False pains* from before back and up in the abdomen (and legs), interrupting the labor-pains. Cramping pains in various parts of the abdomen. Pains spasmodic. *Os uteri round, hard, thick, rigid and undilatable,* and feels as if it would not dilate. Face dark flushed. *Woman stupid and apathetic.* She feels muscular weakness, which arises from weak will power which is unable to command the muscles as when in health. False labor-pains from a few days to weeks before the proper time of labor. *Pains in uterus going through to and up the back.* Sensation of wave from uterus to throat, which seems to impede labor. With every pain the child seems to ascend instead of descending. Nervous chills in the first stage of labor. *Pains insufficient from uterine inertia;* labor-pains gone, os widely dilated, face flushed, she is drowsy and dull. Albuminuria. She dreads beforehand the approaching confinement. Nervous trembling during or just after labor; chatters during first stage. The cervix is soft, flabby; the body of the uterus does not contract at all; there seems to be no attempt whatever at expulsion. Pains start all right, then break and *run up the back,* thus losing their efficacy. Labor-pains extend to the back and hips. Pains tardy. Pains cease on examination because she is "so nervous." Headache during.

ABORTION.—Sharp, distressing pains run *upward,* or *upward and backward.* Loss of will power over the muscles. Confused feeling in the head affecting the mind. Nervous chills. Pain predominates. From sudden depressing emotions with diarrhœa; from fright.

RETAINED PLACENTA.—With cutting pains in the lower abdomen, usually running upward, or sometimes upward and backward, which retards the expulsion.

CONVULSIONS.—She feels and looks stupid. *Preceded* by great lassitude, dull feeling in the forehead, and vertex, fulness in the region of the medulla; *head feels big;* heavy with half stupid look; face red; speech thick. Pulse slow and full. *Head feels large,* or she has a stupefying occipito-frontal headache, with *great muscular prostration.* Albuminuria, with drowsiness, dim vision, and twitching in various parts. *Rigid os uteri* with convulsions, or preceding them, or there may be perfect inaction. Spasms appear early because the os remains hard and thick. Distressing pains from before backward and *upward* in abdomen, though the os may be relaxed and the pulse soft and full. With unconsciousness, labor-pains gone, os widely dilated, great lassitude. Sharp cutting pains that seem to go right through the neck of the uterus, and then upward, with flushed face.

AFTER-PAINS.—Severe pains running *upward,* or upward and backward. With the muscular weakness of the remedy. Severe, and last too long. Sensitive women who cannot compose themselves to sleep. Sleep, with half-waking and murmuring.

GENERALITIES.—Bad effects from great fright or fear. This *fright* is an awe-stricken feeling, deep-seated fright or fear. Loss of sight; double vision; sensation of double vision controllable by the will, during pregnancy; appearance of smoke before the eyes; dim sight. Giddiness and faintness. Drowsiness. Bruised sensation all over the body, as if resulting from severe bodily exertion. Does not wish to be spoken to. Powerless condition of the lower extremities. Respiration frequent and unequal. Fear of death. Vertigo, confusion of head; with loss of sight. Muscles refuse to obey the will when attempting to move. " Wild feeling," alternating with uterine pains. Rushing and roaring in the ears. Face red; yellow; pale, sickly look, dark flushed. Breathing slow, heavy, labored. A peculiar action of the heart, as though it attempted its beat which it failed fully to accomplish, the pulse intermitting each time. Fears that unless constantly on the move her heart will cease to beat. Excessive irritability of mind and body. Yawning, chilly. As soon as she falls asleep, delirious.   Great lassitude, complete muscular relaxation.   Dulness of mind relieved by profuse emissions of urine. Headache commences in the neck quite suddenly, and spreads from thence over the head, or vice versa.

GLONOINUM.

Labor :

Headache during.

HÆMORRHAGE. — Headaches appearing after profuse uterine hæmorrhage.

CONVULSIONS.—Congestive form, with rush of blood to the head. Unconsciousness. Face bright-red, puffed up.   Pulse full and hard. Urine copious and albuminous. After protracted and difficult labor, or instrumental delivery.   Violent throbbing of the heart and carotids.   Froth at the mouth. The hands are clenched, the thumbs being in the palms of the hands ; at other times the fingers spread asunder and are extended. Syncope or sudden fainting, the face being pale or often livid, black spots before the eyes, sudden onset of unconsciousness.

GENERALITIES.—The keynote is: *A tendency*

to sudden and violent irregularities of the circulation. Throbbing headache. Whirling in the head, with giddiness. Great distension of the jugulars. Face deep red; flushed, hot. Effect of sunstroke. *Cannot bear any heat about the head;* can't bear it covered. Cannot endure the heat of the sun or of the stove. Vertigo on assuming an upright position from rising up in bed. Things look strange and unfamiliar. Weeps and shudders between the attacks of pain. Chest feels screwed together; as if laced. Fear. Balancing sensation, constant effort to keep the head erect. Flashes of lightning, sparks, before the eyes. Laborious action of the heart; oppression. Sensation as of expansion of the brain, the head feeling as though it would burst.

GOSSYPIUM.

Labor:

Lingering, almost painless labor, uterine contractions feeble and inefficient. The case presents negative rather than positive symptoms.

ABORTION.—In weakly women. Fœtus comes away, leaving the *placenta in the uterus and the os tightly closed.* Retained placenta after.

RETAINED PLACENTA.—After premature labor, especially. Placenta adheres firmly to the walls of the uterus; no amount of force seems sufficient to dislodge it.

GENERALITIES.—Intermitting pains in the ovaries.

GRAPHITES.

Labor:

In large, corpulent women of venous constitutions, with tettery eruptions, which itch and emit a glutinous fluid. Pains weak, or have ceased entirely.

ABORTION.—

GENERALITIES.—Noises in the ears; can scarcely hear at all in the house, but hears distinctly when riding on the cars or in a carriage. Great dryness of the ears. Exudation of a thin, sticky, transparent, watery fluid from raw or sore places. Tetters in general. Nails brittle and crumbling; deformed; painful; thickening. Changeable mood; sad, thoughts of death; weeping; depressed. Great anxiety. Fretful, irritable; easily vexed. Dizziness. Intolerance of light; light dazzles; flickering before the eyes. Face pale and haggard; pale and bloated; flushed. Tendency to obesity during pregnancy. Nipples painful. Sensation like an electric shock, from heart toward front of neck. Palpitation, with anxiety. Numbness in various parts.

HAMAMELIS.

Labor :

ABORTION.—Much soreness in the abdomen. Hæmorrhage predominates. Discharge continuous; passive; bright-red, not coagulating.

HÆMORRHAGE.—A hammering headache, especially about the temples. Patient exhibits no alarm or anxiety concerning the hæmorrhage. Exhaustion. Varicose veins hard, knotty, swollen, painful. Passive, with anæmia. Flow *steady and slow; dark;* no uterine pains; active; *passive; profuse;* in gushes; red.

GENERALITIES.—Tendency to hæmorrhage, which may come from almost any part. Small loss of blood causes great prostration. Much weariness; *feels so tired.* Bleeding hæmorrhoids, with sense of soreness, weight, and burning. Depressed in mind. Irritable. Swimming sensation on rising. Feeling as if a bolt were passing from temple to temple. Feeling as if both eyes would be forced out of head. Ringing, buzzing in ears. In general uterine hæmorrhage the flow occurs only in daytime, ceases at night.

HELLEBORUS NIGER.

Labor:

CONVULSIONS.—A sharp shock passes through the brain as if by electricity, followed by spasms. Cannot fix ideas; stares; slow to answer; muscles fail to act properly. A noise or a shock shortens the attack.

GENERALITIES.—In dropsical affections. Parts which are usually white turn red. Absence of thirst in all complaints. Chilliness, heat, perspiration without thirst. Urine scanty; coffee-ground sediment. Total unconsciousness. Diminished power of the mind over the body. Delirium. Thoughtless staring. Constantly picking her lips and clothes. Much lamenting and moaning. Sighing. Despairing mood. Irritability, worse from consolation. Thinking about the symptoms lessens them. Throws head back, and from side to side. Pupils alternately contracted and dilated. Roaring and ringing in ears. Face red, hot, but pale; distorted; livid with cold sweat. Gurgling as if bowels were full of water. Spasmodic urging of urine, causing spasms; very little passes. Pulse often slower than the beating of the heart. Arms moving continuously and automatically, except when asleep. Convulsive twitching of muscles.

HELONIAS DIOICA.

Labor:

ABORTION.—Threatened from atonic conditions, especially in habitual abortions; slight overexertion or irritating emotion tends to bring it on. Useful for many of the sequelæ of abortion. From anæmia; from uterine inertia; from ulceration of womb. Discharge coagulated; dark; passive; profuse.

HÆMORRHAGE.—Profuse, dark colored. Flooding on lifting a weight and on least exertion. Face sallow, having an expression of suffering. Pain from the back to the uterus.

GENERALITIES.—In women who are run down as to their nervous system ; who are easily fatigued by any work, and who complain of a tired headache, this tired feeling extending into the limbs. They seem to feel better when working than when first commencing. Urine scanty and turbid. After confinement a tendency to prolapsus and other malpositions of the uterus. Consciousness of a womb. Wants to be let alone ; conversation unpleasant. Fault-finding. Cannot endure the least contradiction. Face pale, earthy. Profound melancholy ; deep, undefined depression. Flooding on lifting a weight. Albuminuria during pregnancy. Nipples tender and sensitive. Backache. Languor. Enervation by indolence and luxury.

HYDROCYANICUM ACIDUM.

Labor :

CONVULSIONS.—*Uræmic convulsions*, with drawing at the nape of the neck from irritation at the base of the brain. Respiration irregular and gasping. Great distress about the heart with weak spells. Surface of the body cold and blue. Excessive prostration. Muscles of the face, jaw, and back are affected. Suddenly a shock is felt, which passes like lightning from head to foot, and then comes the spasm.

GENERALITIES.—Fluids run gurgling into the stomach. Severe prostration, with approaching paralysis of the brain and lungs. Long fainting spells, with palpitation of the heart, and rapid, feeble pulse. Eyes sunken; glossy; blindness. Urine involuntary.

HYDROPHOBINUM (LYSSIN).

Labor:

CONVULSIONS.—The spasms are excited whenever she attempts to drink water, or if she hears it pouring from one vessel into another. Where the sight or sound of water affects her unpleasantly, even though she desires the water.

GENERALITIES.—Irritability. Inclined to be rude and abusive, to bite and strike. Aversion to drinking water, but can take small quantities of chocolate. Large quantities of tough saliva in the mouth, with constant spitting.

HYOSCYAMUS NIGER.

Labor:

Delirium. Startings and jerkings all over face, eyelids, etc.; bluish color of face. *Pains spasmodic;* contracted os uteri. Headache during. Hour-glass contractions. Cold sweat, pale face; face bluish; suffocating spells; jerking and twitching of muscles. Nervous irritability.

ABORTION.—Delirium. Clonic and tonic spasms, rigidity of the limbs. Unconsciousness, or at least loss of sight and hearing, with labor-like pains in the uterine region. Discharge profuse; *bright-red;* continuous.

HÆMORRHAGE.—In women inclined to obesity, with lax muscles and skin; to hysterical subjects, nervous, irritable, excitable, and of sanguine temperament. Great vascular excitement. *With general spasms of the whole body, interrupted by jerks or twitching of single limbs.* Delirium, or even mania. Flow *bright-red, continuous;* pale, with convulsions; worse from every jerk or start of the body in spasms.

RETAINED PLACENTA.—Hour-glass contractions. See under *Labor.*

CONVULSIONS.—With nervous irritability.

Hysterical or epileptic. During spasm limbs forcibly curved and body thrown up from the bed. *Deep sleep with convulsions.* Shrieks, anguish, oppression of the chest, continued delirium or unconsciousness. Bluish face and twitching, and jactitation of every muscle of the whole body, face, eyelids, and all. Spasms followed by paralysis. Retention of the urine. Suffocative spells. With hæmorrhage. After labor hæmorrhage begins with convulsions; every convulsion more blood.

AFTER-PAINS. — With spasmodic pains. Delirium. Much jerking and twitching of various parts of the body.

THE BABY.—Umbilicus open, and urine oozing through.

GENERALITIES.—Marked stupid or drunken look. Face distorted and blue, or swollen or brown red. Sudden starting and jerking of the muscles; one arm will twitch and then the other. Motions are all angular. Often the woman seems to be wild. Frothing at the mouth. Hunger before attacks of convulsions; convulsions following eating. Delirium; in which patient may jump out of bed, throw off the bed clothes, or take off all her clothes and go naked. Nymphomania.

Great restlessness of the body. Spasms in general. Spasms of the eyelids. All objects appear of a red color, or larger. Stupid, or illusions of the imagination and senses. Silly, smiling, laughs at everything, silly expression. Wants to change beds. Scolds; raves. Jealousy. Fright, followed by convulsions. Repeated attacks of fainting. Rolling the head. Staring. Difficult to swallow liquids; attempts to swallow renews spasms. Urine frequent, scanty; difficult from spasms of neck of bladder; has no *will* to urinate; paralysis of sphincter after labor; retention, with constant pressure on bladder; the mother has no desire to urinate though the bladder may be full. Carotids beat violently. Picking fingers; plays with her fingers. Sensation of pricking all over. Want of sensation. She fears she will be poisoned, or betrayed, or injured; she wishes to run away.

HYPERICUM PERFOLIATUM.
Labor :

Labor-pains tardy.

Convulsions.—

After-pains. — Violent, in sacrum and

hips, with severe headache, after instrumental delivery. Burning soreness and sensitiveness of urethra. Retention of the urine.

GENERALITIES.—Bad results from treading on nails, from rat bites, or any punctured wounds; very sore and sensitive to the touch. Delirium; sees spirits, spectres. Anxiety. Melancholy. Removes effects of shock. Sensation as if the head became elongated. Head hot, carotids throbbing. Stares; eyes fixed. Sensation of a worm in throat. Voice has a sharp, unnatural sound. Nervous system much affected. Hard beating of the heart. Spine sensitive and tender. Numbness of left limbs. Weakness and trembling in all the limbs. Injuries to tips of fingers, or other parts rich in nerves.

IGNATIA AMARA.

Labor:

Hysterical symptoms. Pains too weak or ceasing. Rigid os uteri. The labor does not progress. Deep sighs and grief and sadness; she must take a deep breath to breathe at all. Fainting. Much trembling of the limbs. Sobbing.

ABORTION.—Sinking empty sensation in the uterine region. Much sighing and sobbing. Suppressed grief has been the exciting cause. Sensation of "goneness" in the pit of the stomach.

HÆMORRHAGE.—From the abuse of chamomile. Great despondency, sighing, sobbing, etc. From mental excitement and depression. Faint feeling at pit of stomach. Full of suppressed grief.

CONVULSIONS.—The spasms commence and terminate with groaning and stretching of the limbs. Deep sighing and sobbing, with a strange compressed sensation in the brain. Accompanied with vomiting; face unusually deathly pale, especially after fright or grief, night-watching; at times the face may be flushed up. Absence of fever or severe congestion. Head bent backward. In delicate women. Fright with grief the exciting cause; or some violent emotion.

AFTER-PAINS.—Much sighing, sadness, and despondency with the pains.

GENERALITIES.—Especially suited to nervous and hysterical females of mild, but easily excited natures. Suppressed or deep grief, with long-drawn sighs, much sobbing, etc.

8

Unhappiness; entirely absorbed in grief. She wishes for solitude. She will not be comforted. Illusions. Faint, "all gone" feeling in pit of stomach. Hysteria. Changeable disposition. Affectionate. Effects of disappointed love. Convulsive twitching of the muscles of the face or the corner of the mouth. Alternate redness and paleness of the face. Redness and heat of one cheek and ear. Cramp pains in uterus, with lancinations, worse from touching the parts. Desire to take a deep breath. Sighing. Convulsive jerks of the lower limbs. Cracking of the knees. Tingling in the limbs. Spasmodic yawning. Oversensitive to pain. Generally worse from slight touch; better from hard pressure. Headache confined to outside of the head.

IODIUM.

Labor:

Exhaustion. Pulsations in all the arteries at every muscular effort. Great prostration of strength, so that even talking causes perspiration. The sensibility of the nervous system is greatly increased.

HÆMORRHAGE.—With every stool, cutting

in the abdomen, and pain in the loins and small of back. In thin, delicate women subject to corrosive leucorrhœa, with other indica'ions of congested ovaries and uterus. With acute pain in the mammæ. Suitable more especially to chronic menorrhagia.

GENERALITIES.—Very excitable, and nervous or restless, moving about from place to place. Fears that every little occurrence will end seriously. Great dread of people; even of the doctor. Emaciation, even of single parts. Goitre. Extreme hunger; still hungry after eating; eats freely, but loses flesh. Feels constantly as if she had forgotten something. Thoughts fixed. Melancholy mood. Headache as from a tape or band. Convulsive twitching of facial muscles. Violent palpitation. Sensation as if the heart was squeezed. Twitching of muscles. Trembling. *Iodium* should not be given in the lying-in period except in a high potency.

IPECACUANHA.

Labor :

Constant nausea. With each labor-pain a *sharp cutting about the umbilicus darting off to the uterus*, which renders the pain useless. Labor-pains spasmodic, going from left to right. Pains darting, cutting. Clutching about the navel. Faintness.

ABORTION.—*Continuous nausea* without a moment's relief. Cutting pains about the umbilicus going from left to right, passing off into the womb. Labor-like pains. *Continuous, steady, profuse flow of bright-red blood.* Spasms without consciousness. *Hæmorrhage predominating.* Discharge *bright-red; continuous; profuse;* with nausea; with clots, coagulating.

HÆMORRHAGE.—With (or without) incessant nausea and vomiting. Cutting pains about the umbilicus. She is cold and pale, faint, *gasping* for breath, as if panting. Especially after expulsion of the child or removal of placenta. Profuse in *gushes* at every effort to vomit. Faintness. Violent pressure over the uterus and rectum, with shuddering and chilliness. Heat about the head. Complains of dizziness and headache. Debility. Worse when getting out of bed. Coldness of skin which is covered with cold sweat. Hard, labored breathing. Low pulse. So profuse the blood may soak through the bed to the floor, or may run over the foot of the bed. *A steady flow of bright-red blood.* From a dose of *Quinine.* Discharge *constant; profuse; bright-red;* profuse in *gushes;* periodical; with pallor; clotted.

RETAINED PLACENTA.—Deficient labor-pains, with much suffering, but nothing is accomplished on account of the sharp, pinching pain about the navel, running downward to the uterus. Constant nausea. Hæmorrhage of bright-red blood, with retained placenta.

CONVULSIONS.—*Incessant nausea* with occasional spasms. Sometimes rigidity alternates with flexing of the arms and jerking of the arms toward each other.

AFTER-PAINS.—

GENERALITIES.—*A constant but unavailing desire to vomit;* or immediately after vomiting a desire to do so again; *constant nausea.* Suffocative attacks of breathing. Respiration oppressed; anxious; deep, quick; sighing. External coldness. Cold perspiration. Full of desires. Screams, howls violently. Wrapt in thought. Ailments from anger, mortification, or vexation, with indignation.

Vertigo. Face pale; bloated; livid; deathly pale, eyes sunken, and with blue margins; muscular twitchings of face. Attacks of clutching pain in the stomach. Pulse accelerated, but weak. Convulsive twitching of legs and feet. Body rigid, stretched out, followed by spasmodic jerking of the arms. Yawning and stretching. Rash during the lying-in period. Sharp, colicky, pains around the umbilicus, with nausea; clutching and squeezing in the abdomen.

JABORANDI.

Labor:

Tedious labor; normal secretion from the vagina has dried up; passage hot and dry; os unyielding; pains decrease in force.

ABORTION.—

GENERALITIES.—Arrest of heart's action. *Profuse sweat.* Profuse salivation. Great dryness of the mouth. Lachrymation. Contracted pupils. Urging to urinate. Flushing of the face, followed by profuse sweat and acid vomiting. Everything swallowed causes a scraping sensation, from dryness of throat. Thirst.

KALI BROMATUM.

Labor:

CONVULSIONS.—*From pressure of the child on some of the pelvic nerves* or against an undilating os. Pupils dilated, face bright-red, expression of anguish and fear. She is nervous and cannot sleep, must walk about for relief.

GENERALITIES.—Excited, hands constantly busy; timid, suspicious. Imagines she is a devil. Frightful images at night during pregnancy. Delirium with delusions. Melancholy with delusions. Brain irritated, face flushed, pupils dilated, eyes sunken; rolls the head; extremities cold. Sensation as if the bowels were falling out. Twitching of the fingers. Trembling of the hands. Nervous excitement. Great chilliness. Even in a hot room.

KALI CARBONICUM.

Labor:

She is greatly disturbed by *sharp stitching pains.* Sharp cutting pains across the lumbar region, arresting the labor-pains. *She wants her back pressed.* Pains begin in the back, and instead of coming around in front like a regular pain pass off down the buttocks.

Hour-glass contractions. Abdomen bloated with wind. Exhaustion. Restlessness and thirst. She feels the pulsation of all the arteries, even down to the toes. Feeling of emptiness in the whole body, as if it were hollow. The whole body feels heavy and broken down, so that it is only by great effort that she can make any exertion. Pains ceasing, or too weak; insufficient. Bearing down from back to pelvis. Belching with relief. False pains, which usually come in the back and pass down over the buttocks. (Women of sluggish habits.)

ABORTION.—At the second or third months. Weak back. Pain begins in the back and goes down the thighs, or if the pains are more like stitches. Backache when walking. She feels that she must sit or lie down. *Pains predominating.* Pain in the back as if it would break. Labor-like pains, extending into back and thighs. Stitches in renal region. Constipation; stools large and passed with difficulty. From anæmia. Sacculated swelling over the eyes.

HÆMORRHAGE.—*With stitching pains.* Pain in the back extending down over the buttocks. Profuse in delicate anæmic women. Better from eructations; from warmth. At the third month of pregnancy. (Days and weeks after labor.) According to Guernsey, "One of our best remedies for post-partum hæmorrhage."

RETAINED PLACENTA.—Hour-glass contractions. (See under *Labor*.)

CONVULSIONS.—Spasms relieved or passing off by frequent eructations. Does not lose consciousness.

AFTER-PAINS.—*Stitching*, shooting pains. Pains in the back shooting down into the gluteal region or hips.

GENERALITIES.—Frequent chilliness; chilly when out of doors from the least cool air. Throbbing in the bloodvessels all through the body. Local congestions, really anæmic. Complaints following labor. Weakness following labor or abortion, with a troublesome backache. Backache so severe when walking that she feels that she must lie down at once, even in the street, to obtain immediate relief. Startled by imaginary hallucinations, especially from noise if unexpected. Spinal irritation, occurring frequently with uterine symptoms. Pressure as of a weight in the small of the back. Stitching (jerking) pains in *any kind of trouble*. "One of our best remedies following childbirth and its consequences."—GUERNSEY. Headache; stitching, jerking pain. Dazzling of the sight, preventing clear vision; spotted vision. Inactivity of the bowels. Sensation of knocking, or throbbing, or jumping in outer parts Obstructed flatus. Aversion to the open air; despondent in the open air. Generally better from eructations. Sudden attacks of unconsciousness. Absent-minded. Weeps much. Dread of labor (work). Peevish, irritable. Staring. Bag-like swelling of upper lids. Face red and hot; one cheek hot, the other cold; purple; bloated; pale; sickly. Pain in back when swallowing; while or after eating. During pregnancy sick during a walk, no vomiting, feels as if she must lie down and die. Promotes expulsion of moles. Difficult, wheezing breathing. Twitching of muscles. Yawning. Shuddering. Palpitation. Anæmia.

KALI PHOSPHORICUM.

Labor:

Feeble, ineffectual pains. *Tedious labor from constitutional weakness.* Pains weak and irregular. False labor-pains.

CONVULSIONS.—In weak and exhausted women. Oversensitive to all internal and external impressions, with sunken countenance, coldness, and palpitation after the attack. Afraid to be alone. Better by gentle motion.

GENERALITIES.—Morose, irritable. Disposed to weep. Lassitude and depression. Wants to be let alone. Mind sluggish. Feeling as though some dreadful thing was about to happen. Indecision. *Nervous, starts at slightest sound.* Confusion of ideas. Headache from occiput to right eye, through base of brain. Menstrual headache, before and during the flow. Sensation of sticks in the eyes; of sand in eyes; as if they had been full of smoke; as if dry. Rumbling in bowels; flatulence. Urine very yellow. Stitching all through the pelvis and uterus. Bloody discharge during pregnancy. Night pains during pregnancy. Palpitation. Better from belching. Very restless. Very tired feeling. Various itchings.

KREOSOTUM.

Labor:

ABORTION.—At the third month, from metrorrhagia. Hard lump on neck of uterus.

Discharge dark; offensive; intermittent; watery; lumpy.

Intermittent, dark, offensive, corrosive discharge after abortion. Prolapsus uteri after abortion.

HÆMORRHAGE.—Discharge of a large quantity of dark blood; then for a few days bloody ichor with pungent odor, and corrosive itching and smarting of the parts. At the third month. She thinks she is almost well when the discharge reappears. With fainting, pulseless. *Offensive odor of large clots.* Bearing down and weight in pelvis. Sharp stitches darting from the abdomen into the vagina. Blood imprisoned within the cavity of subinvoluted uterus causes gradual dilatation. Flow worse when lying down, stops when rising up. Painful urging toward the genitals. *Scirrhus* of neck of uterus and vagina. Discharge profuse; dark; offensive; pungent; lumpy or clotted; intermittent.

GENERALITIES.—Sorrowful mood; inclined to weep. Morose. Ill-humor. Sick, suffering expression. Face hot, cheeks red, feet cold. Must pass urine when she puts her hands into water, or hears running water. Sudden urging to urinate. Nausea and vomiting during pregnancy. Dragging pain in the back. Yawning. Labor-like pains in the abdomen. Bearing down and weight in pelvis. Violent burning deep in pelvis. Hard lump on neck of uterus. Orifice of uterus wide open, its inner surface like cauliflower. Difficult breathing. Anxiety of the heart. Pain in left hip-joint, as if luxated. Lassitude of all the limbs. Great debility. Fatigue from the least exertion. Loss of sensation; numbness. Putrid leucorrhœa. Tearing pains. Urine offensive.

LAC CANINUM.

Labor:

HÆMORRHAGE.—Blood bright-red, stringy, *hot as fire*, coming in gushes, and clotting easily. Constant bearing-down pains, as if everything would issue from the vulva. Ovarian pains alternating from side to side.

AFTER-PAINS.—Severe pains shooting down the thighs, rather worse on the right side.

GENERALITIES.—Delusion as if surrounded by many snakes. Terror about horrible sights (not always about snakes) presented to her mental vision. Impressed that all she says is a lie. Very restless; cannot control her mind. Depression of spirits;

despondent and hopeless. Very nervous, cursing and swearing. Acute sharp pain, or throbbing, in the head. Constant noise in the head. Excessive dandruff. Sore pimples. Troubles of eyes, ears, nose. Sore throat. Diphtheria, with glistening, shiny, condition of throat; dirty gray membranes; pain and swelling changing sides. Pain on swallowing. Pain and tension in the groins. Pressure and pain in pelvis. Frequent ineffectual urging to stool. Obstinate constipation. Constant desire to urinate; with pain; urine scanty (profuse). Pain in ovaries. Burning sensation in whole uterine region and ovaries. Sharp lancinating pains like knives cutting upward from os, followed by sensation like needles darting upward in uterus. Bearing down as though everything would fall out through the vagina. The labia feel very much contracted. Great swelling of left labia. Strong pulsations in vulva and vagina. Severe retroverted uterus. Burning feet. Face hot, flushed. Breasts sore, sensitive, painful. Galactorrhœa. Knots and cakes in breasts, after miscarriage. Dries up the milk. Dyspnœa. Pains in the chest. Palpitation. Backache. Fœtid sweat in axilla. Sciatica. Various pains in the extremities. Chilliness. Dreams of various kinds of vermin. Much lassitude, weakness. *Pains and disorders of all kinds changing from side to side.* All sores, ulcers, etc., having a shiny, glistening appearance. Pains changing place rapidly. Especially useful in troubles of the breasts.

LACHESIS.

Labor:

Women near the climacteric. Contracted os, with throat and heart symptoms. Fainting; lies as if dead from cardiac syncope, especially when she had previous sadness and gloom; with dread of society. Persistent constipation with sensation as if the anus were closed. Sensitive to touch, especially about the throat.

HÆMORRHAGE.—Paroxysms of pain in the right ovarian region, extending toward uterus, increasing more and more till relieved by a gush of blood.

CONVULSIONS.—Particularly violent in the lower extremities, with cold feet, stretching backward of the body and crying out. Commence on left side and are worse about throat and neck, with trismus and blue face, body bent backward and cold extremities. After the spasm, trembling all over, faint and exhausted. Patient has none while awake, but as soon as she sleeps they appear. Jealousy.

THE BABY.—Cyanosis.

GENERALITIES.—Troubles *beginning* on the left side of any part of the body, *particularly in the throat*. Patient *sleeps into* an aggravation. Blood like *charred straw* in hæmorrhage. Sadness. No desire at all for company. Excessive loquacity, with rapid change of subject. Jealousy. Pride. Suspicion. Restless and uneasy. Burning of the skin ; blueness of. Cyanosis. Delirium. Thinks she is dead. *Cannot bear anything to touch the neck;* general sensitiveness to touch. Tearing pains ; prickling ; pulsating. Chest feels constricted ; stuffed. Palpitation ; anxiety about the heart. Spasms of the legs. Trembling all over ; exhausted, faint. Bearing down pains. Fungus hæmatodes, frequently bleeding.

LAUROCERASUS.

Labor :

HÆMORRHAGE. — Nearly exsanguinated from the loss of blood. She is cold, clammy, pale. Dimness of vision, cold extremities. Peculiar suffocative spells around the heart, gasping for breath, tearing in vertex, stupor or coma. Uterus flabby, or somewhat hard.

CONVULSIONS.—She is conscious of a shock passing through her whole body before the spasm. Much gasping for breath, with blueness of skin. Clonic spasms of all the limbs, with exhaustion and paralytic weakness. Deep, snoring sleep.

THE BABY.—Face blue, with gasping for breath and nearly imperceptible breathing; twitching of muscles of face.

GENERALITIES.—Loss of consciousness, with loss of speech and motion. Insensibility and complete loss of sensation. Fear and anxiety about imaginary evils. Stupefaction. Brain feels loose; or contracted and painful. Objects appear larger. Eyes staring, and wide open. Face sunken, livid; blue; with gasping; bloated. Twitching and convulsions of the facial muscles. Foam at the mouth. Drink rolls audibly through œsophagus and intestines. Pinching about navel. Burning and stinging in and below mammæ. Spasmodic constriction of tracheæ; of chest. Gasping for breath; suffocative spells; dyspnœa. Breathing slow, feeble, almost imperceptible; panting; very difficult. Palpitation. Irregular heart action; pulse very irregular. Ends of fingers and toes enlarged, like knobs. Rapid sinking of the forces; long-lasting faints.

LILIUM TIGRINUM.

Labor:

Neuralgic pains in the uterus. Pains in the ovaries, extending down into inside of thighs. Constant pressure on the rectum with desire for stool: constant pressure on the bladder, with continuous desire to urinate.

AFTER-PAINS.—Neuralgia in and around the uterus. Bloating of the abdomen with the pains a few days after confinement. Smarting in the urethra after urination. Cannot bear even the weight of the covering, as painful parts are very sensitive to touch.

GENERALITIES.—Uterine symptoms following labor and pregnancy. Subinvolution of uterus. The uterus does not regain its normal size after labor. Prolapsus uteri. Heavy, dragging sensation, principally in the hypogastric region. She feels the need of some uterine support.   Urging to urinate, with burning and smarting.   Full, crowded feeling in the chest as though there were too much blood there.   Desires fresh air.   Sharp pain across abdomen from one ilium to the other, with bearing down pains.   Prefers society.   Very low spirited; weeping with feeling of dread.   Crazy feeling in top of head.   Mal-positions of the uterus.   Neuralgic pains about uterus.   Abdomen feels as if it must be supported.   Constant pressure on the rectum.   Constant pressure on the bladder.   Disposed to curse, to strike, to think of obscene things.   Tormented about her salvation.   Irritable; impatient.   Faint feeling, worse in warm room; better in fresh air.   Heart feels as if squeezed in a vise; as if repeatedly grasped, then released; constrictive pain; fluttering.   Aimless hurry and motion.   Weak, trembling, nervous.   Conscious pulsations all over the body.   Whole body feels bruised and sore.

LOBELIA INFLATA.
Labor:

Rigid os uteri and rigid perinæum.   *Violent dyspnœa* with every uterine contraction, which seems to neutralize all expulsive effort. *Thick leathery unyielding cervix*, with (or without) nausea with each pain. Violent pains in sacrum; complains much of her back. *Shooting pains through whole body.* Weakness. Despondency. Sighing. Sobbing.

GENERALITIES. — Desponding; sobbing like a child. Apprehension of death, difficult breathing. Pain through the head in sudden shocks. Violent nausea; with profuse sweat; disappearing very suddenly. Urine deep red color, and deposits a copious red sediment. Violent pain in the sacrum. Sense of great weight in genitals. Morning sickness of pregnancy. Dyspnœa; sense of lump in the throat-pit. Sighing; or a desire to get a deep breath. Shooting pains through whole body, down into tips of fingers and toes. Weakness.

LYCOPODIUM.

Labor:

Spasmodic contraction of the os uteri. Undilated os uteri. During the paroxysms of her pain she is obliged to keep in constant motion; often with weeping and lamenting.

Labor pains go upward or from right to left.
She finds relief by placing the foot against
a support and pressing and relaxing alternately, so as to agitate the whole body.
Pains ceasing; too weak. Retention of urine
due to severe pressure during labor. While
lying in bed she feels as if she would die
from weakness; the lower jaw drops, not
being able to keep the mouth shut. Slow
breathing through the mouth. Eyes half
open, sudden weakness even while sitting.
Red sand in urine. Flatulency.

ABORTION.—Disposition to miscarry. Severe pain in small of back; intolerable before
urinating; with almost entire relief with the
flow. Pain in the uterine region, labor-like,
shooting across abdomen from *right to left*.
Abdomen in constant state of fermentation,
with pains shooting from *right to left* across
the abdomen. Motion of the child excessive
and tumultuous. Feeling of dryness in the
vagina. Weeping; sadness; fainting. Leucorrhœa; itching about vulva. Hæmorrhage.

HÆMORRHAGE.—Profuse, protracted flow;
partly black, clotted; partly bright red;
partly serum; with labor-like pains till she
swoons. Increased flow of blood from va-

gina during passage of hard or soft stool. Cutting across abdomen from *right to left*, with rumbling, discharge of flatus, and better by flow of blood. Sensation as if "full up to the throat."

CONVULSIONS.—An alternate extension and contraction of muscles. Tongue pushed out and withdrawn. Spasmodic trembling of the facial muscles; angles of mouth alternately drawn up and relaxed; alæ nasi alternately expanded and contracted. Fingers extend, then tightly closed. With screaming; foaming at mouth; unconsciousness; throwing the arms about; cardiac anguish.

AFTER-PAINS.—With sticking in the right or left iliac region; dragging toward the inguinal region. Urging to urinate, but inability to do so, with constant bearing down feeling. Retention of urine.

GENERALITIES. — Disposition to be very haughty when sick; mistrustful; peevish; reproachful. Anxious dreams about fatal accidents. Great deal of noisy flatus in abdomen; there seems to be a constant fermentation, which produces a loud croaking sound. Vomiting of sour matter. Clear, transparent urine, with red sandy sediment.

Severe pain in back before urinating, which ceases when urine flows. Pains, or any complaint, *going from right to left. Alternate extension and contraction* of various parts, the skin, sides of mouth, alæ nasi, neck, extremities, etc. Face pale, with circumscribed red cheeks. Flushes of heat in the face. After eating, sudden repletion; drowsiness. Sensation of something moving up and down in abdomen. Cutting across hypogastrium from right to left. Vagina dry. Expels moles. Up and down movement of larynx. Pain from heart to hip and feet when lying down. Intolerance of warm room; better in open air. The whole body feels bruised. Nipples sore, fissured, or covered with scurf; bleed easily. Hard burning nodosities in mammæ, with stitching pains.

MAGNESIA MURIATICA.

Labor:

The labor-pains are interrupted by hysterical spasms. Total insomnia. Constipation. Fainting fits with nausea, better by eructations. Uterine spasms extending to the hips. Twitching, tearing in the hips. Pains ceasing; too weak.

GENERALITIES.—Constipation; stool very difficult, dry, in hard lumps, crumble as they pass the anus; associated with uterine symptoms. After dinner the woman is seized with nausea, eructations, trembling and fainting spells. She is anxious, restless, and always made worse from mental exertion. Congestive headache; sense of boiling water in the cranium; frontal numbness. Sensation as of a ball rising from the stomach into the throat; relieved by eructation. Bearing down in the uterine region, and uterine spasms. Menses black and pitch-like, and are accompanied by pain in the back when walking, and in the thighs when sitting. Leucorrhœa after every stool, or following the uterine spasms. Palpitation of the heart, worse when quiet, better when moving about. Inability to pass urine without pressing down on the abdomen. Tearful, inclined to weep. Tongue feels burnt; mouth feels scalded. Uterine diseases complicated with hysterical complaints. Sense of great fatigue in the legs, even while sitting. Twitching, tearing in the hips. She has many spasms day and night, with great sleeplessness. Formication on the body.

MAGNESIA PHOSPHORICA.

Labor:

Spasmodic labor-pains with cramps in the legs. Excessive expulsive efforts.

CONVULSIONS.—With stiffness of the limbs or of the body; fingers clenched, thumbs drawn in. Insomnia from exhaustion; convulsions worse right side, better by warmth. Staring, open eyes.

GENERALITIES.—The characteristic pains are sharp, cutting, piercing, knife-like; shooting, stitching; lightning-like in coming and going; often and rapidly changing place. Great dread of cold air; of uncovering; of touching affected parts. Pains radiating from the umbilical region. Laments all the time about the pains; sobbing, crying. Sensation as of a strong shock of electricity, passing from head to all parts of the body. Spasms or twitching of eyelids. Menstrual colic. Severe dysmennorrhœa. Neuralgia of the uterus. Chorea; epilepsy; tetanus. Tires very easily, even from talking.

MERCURIUS CORROSIVUS.

CONVULSIONS. — Albuminuria. Excess of

saliva. Trembling or convulsive twitching of the muscles of the face, arms, and legs. Sleepy daytime, wakeful nights. Dull and slow of comprehension. Convulsions of the limbs.

GENERALITIES. — Stares at persons who talks to her. Objects appear smaller; or, double vision. Œdematous swelling of the face, paleness; *albuminuria*. Mouth feels scalded. Convulsive twitchings of the muscles of the face, arms, and legs, and convulsions of the limbs; convulsive contractions. Trembling.

MERCURIUS (Solubilis or Vivus).

ABORTION.—Hæmorrhage, with swelling of the external genitals and inguinal glands. Excrescences on the os; deep ulcers with ragged edges.

HÆMORRHAGE.—Metrorrhagia in aged females. Scorbutic gums, salivation. Mucous, or muco-sanguinolent stools, with tenesmus.

CONVULSIONS.—Much salivation and driveling. Mostly in the extremities. With cries, rigidity, bloated abdomen.

GENERALITIES.—Serious and anxious mental state. Very restless; constantly changing

from place to place. Dread, great anxiety.
Great indifference. Hurried speech. Continuous moaning and groaning. Vanishing
of sight for a few moments. Face pale, yellow, earthy; red and hot cheeks; pale and
sunken; pale, doughy, full. Taste sweetish;
saltish; putrid or slimy. Continual sensation of coldness in the ears. Scorbutic gums;
spongy and bleed easily. Mouth and tongue
moist; much saliva, with thirst. Expels
moles. The *Mercurius* hæmorrhage is profuse, dark and clotted, hanging out of vulva
like icicles; or pale blood. Itching and
burning of the genitals, relieved by washing
in cold water. Jaundice. Deep, sore pain
in pelvis, dragging in the loins. Excrescences on the os, bleeding; deep ulcers, with
ragged edges. Milk in breasts instead of
menses. Dyspnœa. Limbs ache all over;
general soreness. Twitching of arms and
legs. All discharges are acrid.

MILLEFOLIUM.

ABORTION. — Hæmorrhage predominates.
Discharge *bright-red;* profuse. After great
exertion.

HÆMORRHAGE.—Profuse, sudden, *bright-*

red blood. After great exertion, especially in women who are phthisical or subject to hæmoptysis. *Painless* drainage from the uterus, ro pains in the joints. Discharge profuse; *bright-red; constant;* light-colored and fluid; sudden.

GENERALITIES.—Distinguished from *Aconite* by the absence of anxiety and restlessness. May be sad or melancholic. Violent colic, bloody diarrhœa during pregnancy; cramp-like affections during pregnancy. Hot hands and feet. Piercing pains, drawing, tearing. Yawning, without weariness. Rather hæmorrhagic tendency.

MORPHIUM ACETICUM.

Labor:

Excessive pain and uncontrollable nervous irritation. Spasmodic contraction of the os uteri. Extreme susceptibility to pain; pains are so violent as to threaten convulsions, or cause twitching and jerking of the limbs. (Some prefer the Valerianic salt.)

AFTER-PAINS.—Some authorities laud this remedy for after-pains.

GENERALITIES. — We take these two excerpts from Farrington's *Clinical . Materia*

Medica, pp. 247 and 248: " But we may make use of it as a homœopathic remedy. In such violent diseases as cancer Morphia has been successfully given for one of its secondary symptoms, extreme susceptibility to pain; pains are so violent as to threaten convulsions, or cause twitching and jerking of the limbs. Under these circumstances Morphia is a homœopathic remedy. It does not cure, but relieves the pains, not as an opiate by stupefying the patient, but according to the law of homœopathy."

Our *law* is universal; the above symptoms are applicable to all *pain*, whether in cancer or labor or any other trouble. This is homœopathic, and hence the potencies are to be used and not the crude drug.

"I would I had both opportunity and ability to convince the practitioner of the old school of medicine of the absurdity of his indiscriminate use of opiates, and I could hope still more earnestly to dissuade homœopathicians from hiding their ignorance under the anodyne effects of an occasional interpolated dose of morphine or laudanum. The one class ignorant of any other means of assuaging pains, and the other class too lazy to study his case, seek relief for their patients in anodynes. Call them to task for their unscientific practice, and they meet you with the remark, " My duty is to relieve the sick." Let me rejoin, " At any cost? Must you do what you know to be wrong?" "No, but how do you make it wrong?" He then shows the deleterious action of opiates, and asks, " Now, gentlemen, let me ask, is it rational practice to assuage pain with a substance which paralyzes, and so relieves by taking away, *not the disease*, BUT THE ABILITY TO FEEL, THE CONSCIOUSNESS OF SUFFERING." (Italics and small caps, Farrington's.)

MOSCHUS.

Labor :

See Generalities.

CONVULSIONS. — From uræmic poisoning. Stupefying pressure upon the brain. Eyes staring, glistening, pupils dilated ; distension and rumbling in abdomen, with horribly offensive flatus. Urine as clear as water and very copious, or scanty and thick as yeast. Sexual orgasm. Muscular twitching. More tonic than clonic.

GENERALITIES. — Nervous or spasmodic

complaints where the patient feels very cold. Scolding; keeps it up till her lips turn blue, her eyes stare, and she falls to the floor in a swoon. Sudden suffocation from closure of the glottis or cramp of the chest; palpitation. Faint spells, tremulousness of the whole body; coldness of the body; hysterical headache. Fear of death, with pale face and fainting. Vertigo. Nausea. Dim vision. Excited as from alcohol. Raves, speaks rapidly and confusedly. Starts at any noise. Anxiety, with fainting. Faints, with coldness, pale face, full unconsciousness. Muscular twitching. Face wears an expression of surprise. Cries one moment and bursts out in uncontrollable laughter the next. She complains much, but of nothing in particular. Uneasiness in the legs. Hysteria; with fainting or unconsciousness; with coldness of the surface; pale face; suffocative paroxysms; scolding. When the smell of musk affords relief. Great sensation of coldness in outer single parts.

MURIATICUM ACIDUM.

Labor:

Great debility, with hæmorrhoids, so painful that they can hardly be touched, often bleed. So weak that she cannot keep up on the pillow, but constantly slides down in bed.

GENERALITIES.—There may be an appearance of over-strength, but it is in a *weakened* constitution. Exhaustion. Sad and brooding. Unconscious, with muttering delirium. Sighs and groans during sleep. Tongue very dry. Heart irregular and feeble. Pulse intermits at every third beat. Slides down in bed from weakness. Muscular debility following the prolonged use of opium. Cannot urinate without having the bowels move at the same time. *Very tender* hæmorrhoids. Cannot bear the sight nor the thought of *meat*. Affections of the tendo achillis; soles of feet. Restlessness. Tingling, humming, whizzing in ears. Heat in face, glowing red cheeks. Cannot bear least touch, not even of sheet on genitals. Prostration.

NATRUM CARBONICUM.

Labor:

Anguish, tremor, and perspiration with every pain, during which she desires to be gently *rubbed*, which affords her relief. She often says, "Rub me, rub me." Labor-pains weak.

GENERALITIES.—*Depressed and exceedingly irritable*, especially noticed after a meal. Averse to society. Indifference to her own family. Marked degree of gayety. Anxiety, trembling, and sweat during the pains. Emaciation. Great deal of debility caused by the heat of summer, especially when the patient is subject to chronic headache, worse from the heat of the sun. Nervousness or anxiety, worse during a thunder storm. Very nervous from playing on the piano or hearing music. Pressure in hypogastrium. Indurated cervix and ill-shaped os. Painful cracking in region of heart. Twitches and twitching sensation in arms and fingers when taking hold of anything. Cramps of the calves; cutting pain and cramps in the feet. Ankles weak; easily dislocated or sprained. Great debility from any exertion. Aids in expelling moles; prevents false conception.

NATRUM MURIATICUM.

Labor:

Very sad and foreboding. Pains too feeble; ceasing; labor progresses very slowly.

GENERALITIES.—Anæmic women, with thin worn face and general marked emaciation.

Melancholic, easily angered, suffers from nervous weakness, with palpitation, trembling, anxiety, and predominant chilliness. Prolapsed uterus, with backache, relieved by lying on the back or by pressing pillow against back. Feels greatly exhausted from any little exertion of mind or body. Very little exertion produces throbbing all over the body. Sad and tearful. Excitable, laughs immoderately at something not ludicrous. Excitement is always followed by melancholy, anxiety, fluttering at the heart. Cutting in urethra after urination. Headache as of little hammers. Inactive bowels. Enraged when being comforted. Gets angry at trifles. Violent jerks and shocks in the head. Cold sensation on vertex. Buzzing, humming, or ringing in ears. Face yellow; pale; livid; swollen; wan, pasty. Frequent spasmodic closing of the eyelids. Smarting, burning vesicles in mouth and on tongue. Better on an empty stomach. Palpitation. Emaciation even while living well.

NITRIC ACID.

ABORTION.—Labor-like pain in uterine region as if pelvic contents would issue through vulva. Hæmorrhages from uterus in first half of pregnancy from over-exertion, with mental depression.

HÆMORRHAGE.—With violent pressure, as if pelvic contents would issue through vulva; with pain in small of back, through hips and down the thighs. Especially in cachectic women. From overheating; over-exertion; ulcers on os. Discharge dark; bright; profuse; rather fluid.

GENERALITIES. — Usually applicable to dark-haired women. Pricking as from splinters. Sensation as of a band. Sadness, despondency. Fear of death. Imagines her child is not her own. Vindictiveness. Imagines she has a devil in her. Disposition to swear, especially after abuse of mercury. Head very sensitive to rattling of wagons, or to stepping hard. Short of breath. Face pale; eyes sunken. Urine cold when it passes. Pulse irregular; one normal, followed by two small, rapid beats; fourth beat intermits. Excessive physical irritability. Twitching in various parts. Weakness. Cracking in joints. Condylomata or warts. Ulcers with ragged edges; bleed easily. Syphilitic. Cancer uteri. Much swelling of the internal ear.

NUX MOSCHATA.

Labor:

Pains slow and feeble, or suppressed. *Fainting spells.* Very drowsy and sleeping. Pains too weak; *spasmodic and irregular.* Chilly, pale face. Restless. Better when moving about. False labor-pains; women with cool dry skin who never perspire. After delivery, flatulence, with labor like pains; uterus remains uncontracted.

ABORTION.—False labor-pains. Hysterical women disposed to fainting attacks, who greatly dread and fear an abortion. Dry mouth and throat, especially after sleeping. *Hæmorrhage predominates.* Dry skin; want of perspiration. Cramp-like pain in uterine region. Continued and obstinate flooding. Chilliness. From hysteria. Discharge dark and thick.

HÆMORRHAGE. — With dry mouth and tongue; fainting; sleeplessness; hysterical symptoms. Long continued hæmorrhage, especially after abortion. Dark, painless, immediately after delivery. Great fear of death. Flatulent colic, rumbling and distension of abdomen. Expulsion of flatus from uterus and vagina. Uterus remains uncontracted. Discharge dark and thick.

CONVULSIONS.—*Convulsive motion of the head from behind forward.* Hysterical women *who faint easily*, and suffer from great languor in back and knees. Drowsy before and after spasms. Spasms commence with a scream and foaming at the mouth. Labor-pains spasmodic and irregular, or false and weak.

GENERALITIES.—Drowsiness; very sleepy; stupor-like sleep. Chilliness; heat; want of perspiration; no thirst. *Very dry mouth*, tongue adheres to roof of mouth, but no desire for water, rather an aversion to it. Saliva like cotton. Buzzing, humming, or "funny feeling" in body. Delirium, strange gestures, loud, improper talk, sleepless. Laughter, everything seems ludicrous. Changeable mood. Weeping mood. Fickle, irresolute. Brain as if loose, with wabbling motion. Objects look larger; very distant; vanish; red. Blindness, then fainting. Buzzing in ears. Face looks thin; suffering expression. Prolapsus uteri et vaginæ. Violent action of the heart. Disposed to faint; fainting followed by sleep. Small of back and knees feel weak. Numbness in buttocks and down thighs. Fatigue, feels as if she must lie down after least exertion. *Hysteria.*

Feeling as if the teeth were grasped to be pulled out.

NUX VOMICA.

Labor:

Labor-pains entirely or nearly cease. Pains too violent. Extreme pains, apparently constrictive, in the first stage of labor, impeding dilatation of the os. Bruised feeling of abdominal walls or intestines. Each pain attended by sudden sharp cramps in calves of legs; extremities cool. Sensibility to currents of cool air. Irregular pains; labor does not advance; drawing in back and thighs. Pains spasmodic and severe. Every pain causes *vesical* and *rectal* tenesmus and fainting. Headache during. Rigid os uteri. Pains in the loins cause constant urging to stool, with a tendency to rigidity of the os. Great mental depression and nervous irritability. Hour-glass contractions. *Fainting* after eating; after vomiting; after stool; after (every) labor-pain, thereby interrupting the progress of the labor; with congestion of blood to head or chest; with trembling. *Debility* from abuse of coffee, wines, liquors, narcotics, or highly seasoned food; night watching. Cannot sleep after three or four o'clock in the morning. Great sensitiveness to external impressions, noise, talking, strong scents, odors, or bright light. False labor-pains; abdominal spasms; spasmodic pain with urging to stool. *Downward pressure with desire to defecate or urinate.* Pains in the back, and descend thence to buttocks and thighs. Retarded and painful labor in women accustomed to a sedentary life, and those accustomed to high living and an inactive, indolent life.

ABORTION.—False labor-pains with abdominal spasms; spasmodic pains. Pains in the uterine region, *with ineffectual urging to stool or to urinate.* Constipation; large difficult stool, or small and frequent ones. Dyspepsia. Dysuria. Soreness in the uterine region. Very irritable. Dreads to move or to be moved, and feels cross about it. Pains across uterus. *Pain predominates.* From uterine congestion; constipation; stimulants, drugs, or narcotics. Discharge scanty.

HÆMORRHAGE.—With large, difficult stools, or *frequent calls to stool*, with small amount, or none. Bright-red, lumpy, in paroxysms with colic. From abuse of drugs; coffee;

quinine; fright; great exertion; mental excitement or depression; constipation. She leads a sedentary life, high liver. Discharge *profuse; scanty;* bright-red; lumpy; clots.

RETAINED PLACENTA. — Hour-glass contractions. Extreme, constrictive pains impede expulsion.

CONVULSIONS.—Great torpor of the intestinal canal; irritable disposition. From emotions, as anger; from indigestion. Renewed by bright light, sudden jar, noise, or the least touch. Deep sleep following. Opisthotonos, with consciousness. Begins with an aura from the epigastrium.

AFTER-PAINS.—Aching pains. *Sore feeling in the uterine region,* so that she dreads to be moved or disturbed in any way. Irritability. Desires to have the room warm. Desires to be well covered. Every pain produces *desire for stool;* or, sensation of something in rectum to be evacuated. Violent and protracted. Lochia scanty and offensive. Fainting after every pain.

GENERALITIES. — Irritability of a sullen cast; no desire to hold communication with any one; does not wish to be touched. Will scold severely and abuse; maliciousness. An

unsteady, wavering condition of the mind.
Nausea; "If I could only vomit I would
feel so much better." Rumbling in the
bowels; flatulency. Costive; large, difficult
stool. *Constant urging sensation in rectum for
a stool without result, or a scant portion, leaving
a desire as of more to follow.* Yawning, stretching. Chilliness. Face red, feels as if sitting
before a fire. Morning sickness during pregnancy; retching predominates. After lacer-
ated perinæum an internal swelling and burning of the vagina like a prolapsus. Sudden
loss of power in the legs in the morning.
Marked relief from a nap, or uninterrupted
sleep; always worse when the sleep is disturbed. Jaundice. Manner shy and awk-
ward. Thinks she will lose her reason. Time
passes too slowly. Despondent and buoyant
alternately. Stupefaction. Sight blurred by
overheating. Heaviness and contraction of
the eyelids. Ill effects of eye strain. Oversensitive to strong odors. Colic. Hernia.
Painful ineffectual urging to urinate.
Crampy, stitching pains in pelvis; soreness
across pubes. Menses during pregnancy.
Palpitation; on lying down. Sudden stitches
in back when turning, with dull pain while

sitting. Sudden failing of strength. Trembling all over. Tendency to faint. Dyspnœa from upward pressure. Suffering from high living or from a sedentary life. Aggravation in the morning at four o'clock; she is obliged to get out of bed at that time on account of pain in the back, and she finds relief from rising and walking about. She cannot turn over in bed on account of the pain in her back. Pains make her feel cross and morose.

ŒNANTHA CROCATA.

Labor:

CONVULSIONS.—*Uræmic.* Extreme restlessness and anxiety before, and followed by deep coma after the spasm. Rapid convulsive twitching of facial muscles. Face livid and turgid. Hurried, labored breathing. With vertigo, madness, nausea, vomiting, unconsciousness, eyeballs turned up, pupils dilated. *Sudden.* Biting the tongue.

GENERALITIES.—Acts powerfully upon the cerebro-spinal nervous system. Furious delirium. Sudden and complete loss of consciousness. Vertigo, with falling; with nausea, vomiting, syncope, and convulsions. Apoplectic conditions; speechless, insensible; face puffed and livid; pupils dilated; respiration laborious; limbs contracted; trismus. *Rapid convulsive twitchings of muscles of the face. Face livid and turgid;* pale and cold; ghastly; anxious. Foaming at the mouth. Convulsive respiration; hurried, stertorous, short; interrupted by constant sighing. Pulse small, feeble, irregular. *Terrible convulsions*, followed by coma and deep sleep. Bloody froth from mouth and nostrils. Prostration. All symptoms worse from water.

OPIUM.

Labor:
Soporous condition with bloated red face, injected eyes, and stertorous breathing. Twitching and jerking of the muscles. *The bed feels too hot.* Pains suppressed by fear or fright. Pains too weak. Pains cease suddenly and coma sets in between convulsive paroxysms. Retention of stool and urine. With the pains, jerking; twitching; sopor.

ABORTION.—After a great fright. Spasmodic labor-like pains. Pain predominates. *Especially in latter months of pregnancy.* Insomnia with very acute hearing. Constipation.

HÆMORRHAGE.—Restless; the sheets feel too hot to her; she is sleepy, but cannot sleep.

CONVULSIONS. — Suppressed labor-pains may be the proximate cause. Sopor with stertorous breathing, continuing from one spasm to another. Incoherent wandering and convulsive rigidity of the body, with red, swollen, hot face. Hot perspiration. Insensible pupils. Open mouth. From emotions, fright, anger, etc. Begin with loud screams; then foam at the mouth; trembling of limbs; suffocation. *Stupor between spasms.* From heat, or covering up warmly.

THE BABY.—Pale and breathless, cord still pulsates. Spasms; rigidity of the whole body, the trunk curved in the form of an arch.

GENERALITIES.—*Continuous stertorous breathing.* Unconsciousness, eyes glassy, half-closed; deep coma. Imagines part of the body very large. Nervous and irritable. Thinks she is not at her home; this is continually in her mind. Ailments from excessive joy; *fright*; anger; shame. After fright, the fear still remaining. Congestion of blood to the head. On rising, fainting. Dull, stupid, as if drunk. Eyes glassy, protruded, immovable; staring look; red. Face bloated, dark, red, and hot; red; pale, clay-colored, sunken countenance; bluish (purple), swollen. Trembling, twitching and spasmodic movement of the facial muscles. Corners of mouth twitch; distortion of mouth. Foam at mouth. Hernia. Constipation of corpulent, good-humored women. Stool hard, round, black balls. Violent movement of fœtus in utero. Short inspiration; long, slow expiration. Great anguish and dread of suffocation; looks as if dying. Pulse varies. Twitching and spasmodic movement of the arms, hands, and legs. Trembling of limbs after fright. Throws limbs and stretches arms at right angles to body. Faints often. Sighing. Heavy, stupid sleep, with red face. Drowsiness or sopor. Coma vigil. Sleeplessness. *Bed feels so hot she can hardly lie on it.*

PARIS QUADRIFOLIA.

Labor:

AFTER-PAINS. — Intense after-pains, but very imperfect contractions. Entire suppression of lochia, with ineffectual urging to stool. Agonizing headaches, with sensation as if the face were drawn down toward the root of the nose, then backward toward occiput, as if by a string. Eyeballs painful and sore to the slightest attempt at motion.

GENERALITIES.—*Pains as if the eyes were drawn back into the head by strings.* Eyeballs feel too large, and orbit too small. Headache of spinal origin, which arises from the nape of the neck and produces a feeling as though the head were immensely large. Headache aggravated by close thinking. Great sensitiveness to offensive odors. Feels very large in size. Urine with greasy cuticle on the surface. Loquacious mania. Silly conduct.

PHOSPHORUS.

Labor :

Pains distressing and of very little use. Very weak and empty feeling in abdomen, sometimes with cutting pains. Pains in sacrum after labor. In tall, slender women of phthisical habit.

ABORTION. — Great weakness in uterine region. Pulsating, burning pain in vertex, worse on forehead, nausea and vomiting; from morning till noon. Stool long, narrow, dry, and difficult. Profuse and long-lasting flow of blood. Tall, slender women.

HÆMORRHAGE. — After difficult labor, in tall, slim, phthisical women. Constipation. During pregnancy. Pouring out freely, and then ceasing for a short time. Weeping and sad mood. Painful feeling of *weakness* and sensation of *coldness* or *emptiness* across the whole abdomen. Abdomen very sensitive, painful to touch. Small of back *pains as if broken;* a dragging; worse laughing or moving. Discharge profuse, long lasting. The characteristic constipation. Feeling of intense heat running up the back.

CONVULSIONS.—*Previous to the convulsion a sensation of heat rushes up the back into the head.*

AFTER-PAINS.—Pains in the sacrum after labor.

GENERALITIES. — Exceedingly susceptible to external impressions; can bear neither light, sounds, nor odors; very sensitive to the touch. Stupor; delirium. Hysterical alternation of laughing and weeping. Melancholy. Easily angered. Nervous vertigo; or from abuse of narcotics or coffee. Dandruff. Difficult hearing, especially for the

voice.   Sounds reverberate.   Face pale;
ashy; livid; bloated, lips blue; hippocratic.
Menorrhagia in nursing women.   A very *weak,
empty, or gone sensation*, felt in the *whole abdominal cavity.*   Vomiting as soon as *food* or
drink becomes *warm in the stomach.*   Sensation of *heat* or *burning in the back, between the
shoulder-blades.*   Wants cold food and drink.
Constipation; fæces slender, long, dry, tough,
and hard, like a dog's.   Nymphomania.
Stitches upward, from the vagina into the
pelvis.   Oppression and anxiety in the chest.
Noisy, panting breathing.   Difficult inspiration.   Palpitation from every motion.
Back pains as if broken.   Twitching of the
feet.   Frequent fainting; pale, cold; sudden
syncope, lying as if lifeless.   Burning and
stinging in the skin.   Much belching of wind
after eating.   Feeling of intense heat running
up the back.   All objects appear to be covered with a gray veil.   Suitable especially
for tall, slender women.

PLATINA.

Labor:

Labor-pains interrupted by the very painful *sensitiveness* of the vagina, external parts,

and the os uteri. Spasmodic, very painful, inefficient pains. Pains too weak. Her thoughts horrify her. Hour-glass contractions; severe cramping pains in the uterine region; oozing of dark grumous blood. *Labor-pains all on left side*, painful, spasmodic, ineffectual. Weeps with her pains. Much anguish. After labor, so sensitive, she cannot bear the touch of the napkin.

ABORTION.—Labor-like pains in the uterine region. Tremulous sensation from vulva into the abdomen. Mons veneris and vulva feel cold and sensitive to the touch. Discharge black; thick; coagulated; dark; fluid.

HÆMORRHAGE.—Pain in the back extending into both groins, and *excessive sensibility of the genitals*. Sensation (with flowing) *as if the body were growing larger* in every direction. Clots hard and black, mixed with fluid blood passing away in a dark tarry appearance. Dark painless hæmorrhage. During pregnancy. Great sexual excitement. Her thoughts horrify her. Discharge dark; thick; black clots; fluid; one thick, black tarry mass; thick black, not coagulated.

RETAINED PLACENTA.—Hour-glass contractions. Very great sensitiveness of the parts;

severe cramping pains in the uterine region. Constant oozing of dark grumous blood from the vagina.

CONVULSIONS.—From nervous excitement, preceded or followed by constriction of œsophagus and respiratory embarrassment, sometimes sudden arrest of breathing. Spasms alternating between convulsive actions and opisthotonos. In women having profuse, dark menses, and are proud and haughty. Spasms alternating with dyspnœa and suffocation. Twitching of single muscles, trembling, shivering.

GENERALITIES.—Hysteria. The patient is very haughty, looks with disdain upon every one and everything. Sensation of dread and horror. Past events trouble her. Her thoughts horrify her. *Nymphomania.* Cramping pains in inner parts, muscles, joints, etc. Gnawing pains in outer parts. Sensation of a hoop around parts. Violent shocks as if from pain. Sensation of cold in outer parts. Worse from smell of flowers; cannot endure them. Thoughts of death horrifying; any serious thought is terrifying. Everything seems strange and horrible to her. Thinks all persons are demons. Mania, with great pride; fault-finding; unchaste talk. Imagines every-thing around her is small and every one in-ferior to her in mind and body. Low-spirited; **inclined** to tears. Weeps with the pains. **Much anguish.** Indifference. Sen-sation of **water** in the forehead. Sensation of coldness in the eyes; in the ears; in the mouth. Ringing, rolling, or rumbling sounds in the ears. Face pale, sunken; red and burning hot; sense of coldness. Jac-titation of muscles in region of stomach. Constipation; stool like putty, adheres to rectum and anus. Induration of uterus; ulceration. Voluptuous tingling in vulva. Difficult breathing. Spasmodic affections of hysterical women. Tetanic-like spasms, with wild shrieks. Violent yawning. Pains increase and decrease gradually. Sweat only during sleep. Dark hair; rigid fibre.

PLUMBUM.

Labor:

ABORTION.—*Tendency to abort from non-de-velopment of the uterus.* The fœtus grows, but the muscular fibres of the uterus do not de-velop in proportion, hence the uterus is no longer able to accommodate the growing fœtus and abortion ensues. Pain drawing from abdomen to the backbone, as if the abdomen were drawn upward by a string, making the abdomen concave rather than convex. From lead poisoning. Constipation, stool in balls. Much depression of spirits.

HÆMORRHAGE.—With the sense of a string pulling from the abdomen to the back. Constipation, fæces composed of lumps packed together like sheep's manure. Anxiety about the heart. Skin dry, pale, yellowish. Melancholic mood. Dark clots alternating with fluid blood or bloody serum. Worse from motion.

GENERALITIES.—Drawing pain from before backward, as though the abdomen were drawn in and through towards the backbone, sometimes making the abdomen concave. Sensation as though a string were drawing the abdomen in. Generally there is great despondency with this pain. Jaundice. Terrible colic. Retraction of soft parts in general. Convulsions, with jerking. Wild delirium, with distorted countenance. Melancholy. Depression of spirits. Eyeballs feel large; lids spasmodically contracted; paralysis of upper lids. Face pale; yellowish, like a corpse; bloated; greasy, shining. Constipation; with the retraction of the abdomen, and with marked spasm or contraction of the sphincter ani. Urging to stool, with sensation as though a string were drawing the anus up into the rectum. Abdomen very hard. Constriction in throat; sense of plug in throat; wants to stretch limbs during ovarian pains. During pregnancy, feeling as though there was not room enough in abdomen; or a peculiar sensation, at night in bed, which causes her to stretch violently for hours together; feels that she *must* stretch in every possible direction. Dyspnœa. Pulse variable. Convulsive motion of arms and hands. Cramps in calves. Paralysis. Epilepsy.

PODOPHYLLUM PELTATUM.

ABORTION.—Pain predominates. Pain in the ovarian regions, especially at night, disturbing sleep, making her nervous and restless; this condition may occur night after night and finally induce miscarriage. Prolapsus uteri (especially after abortion and confinement), the womb falls very low, painfully so. Pain in the uterine region, laborlike, extending into the ovarian region. Prolapsus uteri from overlifting or straining. Prolapsus ani with stool.

HÆMORRHAGE.—From *straining or overlifting*. Prolapsus uteri et ani. Constipation.

AFTER-PAINS.—With strong bearing-down pains. With heat and flatulency.

GENERALITIES.—In many troubles of pregnant females; weak, bearing-down sensation, in the abdomen after parturition, with sensation as if the intestines were falling down; prolapsus uteri with pain in the sacrum. Diarrhœa after eating or drinking. Prolapsus of the rectum after stool. Feels fatigued; depressed. Sallow complexion. Pendulous abdomen, after confinement, with much nervous irritability and sleeplessness; feels weak and unable to move about. Subject to "bilious attacks." Numb aching in region of left ovary; heat down thigh; third month of pregnancy. Sensation as if the genitals would come out during stool. Prolapsus uteri from overlifting or straining. Swelling of the labia during pregnancy. During pregnancy can lie comfortably only on stomach. Inclined to breathe deeply; sighing. Palpitation. Sudden shocks of jerking pains.

PULSATILLA.

Labor:

Uterine inertia. Pains ceasing (from hæmorrhage or otherwise); distressing; spasmodic; irregular; too weak; too strong; too slow; ineffectual; exciting fainting. Pains excite palpitation, suffocating and fainting spells; she must have doors and windows open. No thirst, very slow labor. Chilliness and pale face. Hour-glass contractions in very mild, tearful women. False pains. *Labor-like pains which make her walk about* to obtain relief: she cannot sit long at a time. She weeps and frets and fidgets, and is very despondent. She complains that the child "lies so queer," and pains her so that she cannot lie on her back. Soreness of the uterus and abdominal walls. Drawing, pressive pains extending toward the uterus, with qualmishness. Contractive pains in the left side of the uterus, like labor-pains, obliging her to bend double. Violent cutting pains low down in the abdomen, with a sensation as if a stool would occur. Cutting, dragging pains in the hypogastrium, extending around to loins, and making her feel faint. Pains worse in the back; with no progress. *Abnormal presentations* may be righted if given before the membranes are ruptured or the presenting parts are firmly engaged. (This has been verified by the best prescribers.) Suitable for mild, tearful women, who are in an apparently healthy condition, yet the uterus seems almost inactive. (Give *Puls.* high for prompt success with any symptom.)

ABORTION.—Black blood passed with labor-pains. Pains and hæmorrhage alternate. Pains predominate. Pain in uterine region. Discharge arrested for a little while, then it reappears with redoubled violence; this *cessation and renewal are often repeated.* Cannot endure a close or warm room, and wants air. From anæmia; from cold or damp; from uterine inertia. Discharge intermittent; black and coagulated; black, in gushes; bright-red, in gushes; dark; in gushes; coagulated.

HÆMORRHAGE.—Intermittent black, with clots, *alternating with labor-pains.* Dark clots in paroxysms. Ceases for a few moments, then recommences with redoubled force. Most profuse in persons given to reveries. In mild, gentle, weeping women, who want plenty of fresh air by having doors and windows open. From a dose of Quinine; from retained placenta; from coagula. Discharge intermittent; dark; clotted; thick; or thin, watery; changeable in character; profuse.

RETAINED PLACENTA.—With intermitting hæmorrhage. Retention of urine with heat, redness and soreness of the hypogastrium externally, which is painful to touch. Hourglass contractions in mild, tearful women. Want of expulsive power. Inertia uteri. Adherent. In mild, tearful women; inclined to weep because her labor is not completed. Desire for fresh air. Very restless. "This remedy is more frequently indicated and more generally useful than all others." —GUERNSEY.

CONVULSIONS.—Following deficient, irregular, and sluggish labor-pains. Countenance cold, pale, and clammy. Loss of consciousness and motion. Stertorous breathing and full pulse. Mild and tearful women who want fresh air when conscious.

AFTER-PAINS.—The pains become worse toward evening. Thirstlessness. Bad taste in the mouth. Restlessness. Changeable feeling, now better, then worse. Too long. Mild, tearful women who want fresh air. She feels uncomfortable if the room be warm, and complains of its warmth.

GENERALITIES.—Pains constantly change their location, flying from one part to another; sometimes existing with intense severity, then suddenly becoming very mild, and *vice versa.* In women of a mild, yielding, or good-natured disposition; or in those *very easily excited to tears* (or laughter)— they are apt to burst into tears when spoken to, or when they attempt to give their symptoms, etc. *Cannot breathe well in a warm room;* better from fresh open air. Religious mania; sees the devil coming to take her. Dread of men. Anguish. Envy; covetousness. Headache, worse in a warm room. Eyes oversensitive to light. Eyes feel as if covered with a mist. Ears feel stuffed up. Flushes in the face. Throat sore. Thirstlessness. Chilliness. Dyspnœa. Vertigo. Burning in region of the heart. Violent palpitation. Knees inflamed, swollen. Legs

worse hanging down. Hysteria; symptoms
ever changing. Fainting fits, great paleness
of face; shivering, coldness. Violent trembling all over. Yawning. Pains appear
suddenly, leave gradually. Pains cause her
to move about for relief. Pains are better
from cold food, drink, or air. Pulsations
through the whole body. Varicose veins.
Difficult breathing. Expels moles.

PYROGENUM.

Labor:

ABORTION.—With bright-red blood, with
dark clots. In the course of septic or zymotic diseases. From la grippe.

HÆMORRHAGE.—Of bright-red blood, with
dark clots. Pyrogen resembles *Ipecac.* very
closely in uterine hæmorrhage; if Ipecac.
fails when seemingly well indicated, think
of Pyrogen.

CONVULSIONS.—

GENERALITIES.—*A very rapid pulse, without
corresponding increase of temperature. Pulsations felt all through the body, head, ears,* etc.
Painless pulsations. Aching all over the
body and extremities. *Great restlessness*; can
lie in one position but a very short time;

better when first beginning to move. *Bed feels very hard.* Worse from sitting up in bed; from rising up. Amelioration of the death-like restlessness from sitting up in chair and rocking hard. Very loquacious. Irritable. She feels when lying on one side that she is one person, when lying on the other side that she is another person. Sense of being crowded with arms and legs. Face pale; very red; yellow; circumscribed redness of the cheeks. Terribly foetid taste. Tongue fiery red; glossy, shiny; very dry, but easily moistened. Stool, urine, perspiration, menses, etc., all horribly offensive. Pain starts in the umbilicus or a little above, and passing down toward the uterus, midway meets a similar pain from the uterus towards the umbilicus, then gradually dies out, to be repeated. *In septic poisoning after abortion or confinement* this is the remedy par excellence.

RHUS TOXICODENDRON.

Labor:

Occasional paroxysms of pains extending down the posterior surface of the limbs. Great restlessness, with relief for a short

time from change of position. Must change
position quite often. Fainting. Exhaustion. Cold water disagrees. Hour-glass
contractions.

ABORTION.—From a *wrench, strain, a misstep, lifting or overexertion;* from shocks, falls,
concussions; from rheumatism. Pains at
night, especially in the latter part. She is
restless. Cramps in the legs. Drawing
pain in the back. Pain predominates. Discharge intermittent ; bright-red.

HÆMORRHAGE.—From a *strain or wrench;
false step; lifting.* In rheumatic women,
worse on change of weather. With labor-like pains. Discharge bright-red ; lumpy,
or clots; in paroxysms with colic.

RETAINED PLACENTA.—Hour-glass contractions; paroxysms of pain extending
down posterior surface of the limbs. Restless, with relief from change of position.
Must change position often.

AFTER-PAINS.—Come on one after another,
and sometimes last all night. Frequent
change of position gives relief for a time.
Pains worse at night with great restlessness ;
at times they last all night, without much
pain during the day. Likes a warm room

and plenty of covering. Cramps in the calves.

GENERALITIES.—An irresistible desire to move, or *to change the position frequently, with temporary relief;* usually worse at night. Painful stiffness when *first beginning to move;* better from *continued* motion. Any trouble *resulting from a sudden and thorough wetting by a shower of rain;* by getting wet in any way. Must change her position frequently at night, with temporary relief. Stupefying headache. Brain feels loose. Photophobia. Face fiery red; pale, sunken. Fever blisters around the mouth. Throat constricted. Nausea. Bearing down, when standing or walking; prolapsus uteri from over-exertion or lifting; backaches, feeling better by lying on something hard. Discharge of blood during pregnancy. Palpitation violent when sitting still. Spasmodic trembling in limbs when stepping out. Cramps in legs and feet, must walk about. Spasmodic yawning.

RUTA GRAVEOLENS.

Labor :

Lame and sore all over. Very weak, feeble

contractions. Prolapsus ani after. Pains ceasing.

ABORTION.—Metrorrhagia as a forerunner. *Miscarriage of dead children at about the seventh month,* followed by a long and slow recovery. Corrosive leucorrhœa.

GENERALITIES.—Injuries of the periosteum, causing a bruised sensation. The rectum protrudes from the anus after confinement. Prolapsus ani, may come down on attempting, or after every stool. Pain in the bones and outer parts as if bruised. Painfulness of the bones in general. Gnawing in the inner parts. Aggravation from looking fixedly at an object. Short breath, with tightness of the chest. Anxious palpitation. Painful spot on sternum; below right scapula. Tottering as if the thighs were weak; limbs pain when walking. Itching of the skin after eating meat.

SABINA.

Labor:

Pain felt all the way between the sacrum and the pubes, from one to the other—not particularly in front or behind, but right along from the sacrum to the pubes.

ABORTION.—At or about the *third month.* Pains commencing in small of back and going around and through the pubes. Violent forcing or dragging or drawing pain extending from the back directly through tò the pubes. Hæmorrhage predominates. *Profuse bright-red or dark fluid and clotted discharge.* Pain in uterine region with faint, sick sensation in abdomen. Labor-like pains in uterine region. Bright-red, clotted flow, *worse with every motion,* followed by a flow of dark-red clotted blood. Painless loss of dark-red blood, after. From hysteria; uterine inertia; plethora. Discharge black, coagulated; dark; *bright-red,* coagulated; continuous; offensive, or fœtid; in gushes; *profuse;* intermittent; watery; *worse from motion;* pale; very thin.

HÆMORRHAGE.—Forcing down pain from sacrum to pubes. The *slightest motion increases the flow,* but walking about diminishes it. Dark-red flux, with very *dark clots in thin watery blood.* (More frequently bright-red blood). Painless dark hæmorrhage after delivery or abortion. *Equal parts of clotted or fluid, dark or bright flow.* Pain or uncomfortable feeling between the sacrum and pubes. Frequently attended by pains in the joints. Great weakness or nervousness in head and extremities. After leucorrhœa. Discharge *profuse;* clotted, coagulated; *bright-red; dark-red;* pale; offensive.

RETAINED PLACENTA.—Pain or uneasy bad feeling from sacrum to pubes. A slight sensation as of motion in the abdomen. *Intense after-pains, notwithstanding the retained placenta,* with discharge of fluid blood and clots in equal parts, with every pain.

AFTER-PAINS.—Pains run from sacrum to pubes. With every pain (usually severe) discharge of fluid and clotted blood. At times pains from back and sacrum to thighs. Abdomen very sensitive to touch.

GENERALITIES.—The characteristic *pain all the way from the sacrum to the pubes. The blood is in fluid and clots together*—the liquid blood will flow, then will come a clot, and the blood may be flowing rapidly. Better from exhalation; worse from inhalation; taking a deep breath. Shortness of breath. Music intolerable, and aggravating. Buzzing in the ears. Face pale; eyes lustreless, with blue rings around them. Flushes of heat in the face, chilliness all over, and coldness of hands and feet. Stitches in the stomach extending to the back. Labor-like pains in abdomen down to groins. Pressing down toward the genitals. Slight sensation of motion in the abdomen, as if something were alive. Menses too profuse. Stitches from below upward, deep in vagina. Promotes expulsion of moles. Tendency to abort at or about the third month. Palpitation at every motion, especially when ascending. Pulse unequal. Drawing, tearing pains in extremities. Lassitude and heaviness. Fig-warts.

SECALE CORNUTUM.

Labor :

Irregular, weak, suppressed *or* very distressing pains ; uterus flabby. Pains distant or ceasing. Fainting fits. Hour-glass contractions ; a sensation of constant tonic pressure in the uterine region, prolonged bearing down and forcing pains, causing great distress. Wants fresh air. Don't like to be covered. The strength of the uterus weakened by too early or perverted efforts, sometimes a few weeks before regular labor

THERAPEUTIC INDICATIONS.   179

sets in. *Everything seems loose and open, without action.* Prolonged, but ineffectual pains. Bearing down in the sacral region, a sort of prolonged urging in the abdomen. False pains, with bloody discharge. Especially in weak, cachectic, scrawny, women, with sallow complexion, or in those debilitated from venous hæmorrhage or by *frequent and repeated child-bearing.*

ABORTION.—Especially at *the third month.* In feeble women who have borne many children, or of the usual cachectic constitution. Copious black fœtid fluid discharge. Convulsive movements. Hæmorrhage predominates. Labor-like pains in the uterine region alternating with hæmorrhage. Difficult contractions of the uterus after abortion. Tingling all over the body, better by having the limbs rubbed. She *holds her fingers spread apart*, which seems to bother her more than the flowing. Wan, sunken countenance, pulse almost extinct, fear of death. False labor-pains, with bloody discharge. Followed by tearing pains in the limbs. From anæmia ; passive uterine congestion ; uterine inertia. Discharge black ; foul-smelling clots ; offensive ; coagulated ;

fluid; bright-red gushes; profuse; watery; worse from motion.

HÆMORRHAGE.—Passive, of dark, fœtid, thin blood, in feeble cachectic women who have borne many children, or have resided for a long time in tropical climates. With strong and very painful bearing down pains before the flow. Desire for fresh air. General coldness, while she feels too warm and does not want to be covered. Prostration. From fright during pregnancy. Painless flooding. Feverish pulse. Formication or tingling all over the body and a desire to have her limbs rubbed, followed by unconsciousness and a cold condition. She is bothered because she seems impelled to hold her fingers apart. From retained placenta with delirium, loquacity, etc. From uterine atony, especially after protracted labors. Discharge continuous; *passive*; *profuse*; *worse from motion*; black liquid; brown liquid; large black clots; dark fluid; fœtid or offensive; persistent; bright-red and intermittent.

RETAINED PLACENTA.—Constant sensation of bearing down; it seems to her to be too constant and strong to be effectual. Passive hæmorrhage. The parts seem relaxed and there is absence of uterine action. Irregular hour-glass contractions. Wishes for fresh air. Don't want to be covered, distressed by warmth. Pains cause great distress. Especially after miscarriage. Pains very imperfect, or else there is a prolonged tonic contraction. In tall, scrawny women.

CONVULSIONS.—Violent forcing pains. Pains irregular, weak. Opisthotonos, hands stretched out, cramps in calves of legs. Fainting fits. Labor ceases, and twitchings or convulsions begin. Retained placenta. In scrawny, poorly nourished women with feeble labor-pains. "Ergotismus convulsivus." With hæmorrhage.

AFTER-PAINS.—In elderly women *who have borne many children* and are thin and scrawny. Labor-like pains frequently repeated, which are tonic, prolonged, pressing and forcing. Thin, brown lochia. Lochia offensive. Although she feels cold she prefers *not* to be covered. Post-partum conditions of primiparæ.

GENERALITIES.—She may have mania, during which she laughs, claps her hands above her head, seems to be beside herself.

Especially suited to the thin, scrawny, wrinkled women, and in those who have borne many children. She is cold, but she does not wish to be covered up. Copious vomiting cf a mixture of thick, black, pitchy, bilious and slimy matter. Vertigo ameliorated by rocking. Crawling on the skin as of insects. Great anguish. Wild with anxiety. Fear of death. Delirium. Mania. Giddiness. Unconsciousness, with deep sleep, preceded by tingling in head and limbs. Photophobia. Eyes feel as if spasmodically rotated. Eyes sunken, surrounded by blue margin. Eyes looked fixed, wild, glazed. Face pale; pinched; dark-red and swollen; wan, fearful countenance; tingling in face. Muscular twitchings, usually commence in face and then spread all over the body, sometimes increasing to dancing and jumping. Spasms of the tongue. Arrested development of the fœtus. During pregnancy frequent and prolonged forcing pain, particularly in thin, ill-conditioned women; cramps in calves. Lochia dark, very offensive; scanty or profuse. Respiration slow; labored and anxious; oppressed. Pulse often unchanged during violent attacks;

generally slow and contracted; intermittent. "Kink" in the back. Violent pains in the finger tips. Cramps in calves; in fingers and toes. Tingling in toes. Lassitude, heaviness, trembling of limbs. Limbs cold, covered with cold sweat. Spasmodic twitchings. Irregular movements of the whole body. Frequent yawning. Formication under the skin. Burning in all parts of the body, as if sparks were falling on them. Sensation of coldness in abdomen and back; horripilation in abdomen, back and limbs. Generally better from being uncovered and from cold. Should never be given in material doses.

SEPIA.

Labor:

Induration of the cervix; rigid os uteri in consequence. Shooting, darting, needle-like pains, extending upward from the neck of the uterus. Spasmodic contractions of the os uteri. Shuddering attends the pains. She wants to be covered up more, as she thinks she can endure the pains easier. Pains ceasing. Pains distressing. Pains spasmodic. Pains too weak. Hour-glass contractions, with the little darting pains, shooting upward from the cervix. Flushes of heat. Cold hands and feet. A distressed empty feeling in the pit of the stomach. Fainting. False labor-pains; frequent bearing-down pains in the back and abdomen; she crosses her legs to relieve them. Sense of weight in the anus as from a heavy ball. Dyspnœa. Weak feeling in the abdomen.

ABORTION.—Habitual from the fifth to the seventh month. Irritable nerves and laxness of tissue, with evidence of disturbed circulation. *Sensation of weight in anus like a heavy ball*, with constipation. Painful, empty, gone, sensation in the pit of the stomach. The fœtal movements are very feeble, scarcely perceptible. Yellow spots on face; yellow saddle across nose. Pain predominates. Colicky pain in the uterine region. Labor-like pain in the uterine region as if the pelvic contents would issue through the vulva. Fulness and pressure of blood to head and chest. Sense of heaviness in abdomen. Flushes of heat, with faintness and momentary attacks of blindness, especially in a warm, close room.

From uterine congestion; from indurated cervix; from leucorrhœa.

HÆMORRHAGE.—Plethora, or congestion with sensation of weight. Pain in right groin. Fine darting pains in cervix from below upward. Feels better from drawing up the limbs. Yellow spots on face; yellow saddle across nose. Icy-cold paroxysms and flushes of heat; cold feet. Painful, empty, gone feeling in pit of stomach. Urine fœtid and has sediment as if clay were burned on bottom of urinal. Constipation. Sense of weight in anus. From least cause. Chronic congestion of uterus with sense of weight as if all would come out of vulva.

RETAINED PLACENTA.—Little, sharp-shooting pains in the cervix, sometimes with burning. Hour-glass contractions. Flushes of heat. Cold hands and feet. *Where no symptoms are present, after abortion.*

AFTER-PAINS.—Constant sensation of weight in anus as of a ball. Pain shooting upward in vagina. Pains felt mostly in back, severe forcing or bearing down occurring in paroxysms in the back.

GENERALITIES.—She is very uneasy about the state of her health; constantly worrying, fretting and crying about her real or imaginary illness. Great indifference. Fits of involuntary weeping and laughter. Is easily offended. Involuntary jerking of the head. Great sensitiveness to odors. Prolapsus uteri; of the vagina; with constipation. Induration of the neck of the uterus. Metrorrhagia during pregnancy, especially fifth and seventh month. Soreness of abdomen of pregnant women; feel the motion of child too sensitively. Oppression of chest and shortness of breath when walking. Palpitation after emotions of mind. Sensation as of running of a mouse in limbs. Restless, fidgety. Hysterical spasms. Sensation of a ball in inner parts. Tingling in outer parts. Excessive sensitiveness to pain. Ringworms. The usual *yellow saddle across the bridge of the nose*. Painful sensation of emptiness in the stomach. Smell of food repulsive.

SILICA.

Labor :

ABORTION.—Hæmorrhage after. Spinal affections. Constipation or difficult defecation, as if the rectum had not power to expel the fæces, and when the stool recedes, pressing-down feeling in the vagina. Parts tender to touch.

HÆMORRHAGE.—With the characteristic stool. Terribly offensive sweating of the feet.

GENERALITIES. — Screaming violently. Over-anxious about herself; low-spirited; gloomy, feels as if she would die. Cannot bear to think. She is constantly occupied with pins—counts them, hunts for them, etc. Cold feeling from nape of neck to vertex. Shooting from nape to vertex. Ringing or roaring in ears. Face pale; cachectic; yellow; distorted. Stool large, composed of hard lumps; expulsion difficult; recede after being partly expelled. Metrorrhagia, offensive foot-sweat; icy-cold body; painful piles. Bloody discharge between periods. Promotes the expulsion of moles. Hard lumps in the mammæ. Arrest of breathing when lying on back; when stooping. Cannot take a long breath. Palpitation while sitting; violent hammering palpitation after quick or violent motion. Restless, fidgety; starts from least noise. Trembling in all the limbs. Want of animal heat. Feels as if divided into halves and that the left side did not belong to her. Pricking-tingling in various parts. She is always worse during the increase of the moon.

STANNUM.

Labor:

Spasmodic labor-pains. The pains seem to exhaust her very much and make her speech difficult from weakness in the chest. She cannot answer questions; she is all out of breath; the labor does not progress. Sense of weakness in the larynx and chest, thence all over the body, from talking or reading aloud.

GENERALITIES.—Usually sad and weeping. Crying usually makes her feel worse. *Low-spiritedness in lung troubles.* She is nervous and weak; so nervous, irritable and weak she becomes anxious and has palpitation of the heart from very little exertion; can scarcely move about. She feels that she could not walk down stairs, her limbs feel so weak. Odor of cooking causes vomiting. Weak, gone feeling in the stomach. Prolapsus of the uterus or vagina. The limbs feel as heavy as lead. Weakness of the limbs, worse when descending or assuming a sitting posture. So weak that she must drop down suddenly, but can readily get up. Trembling of the arms and legs. Weak, gone feeling in the chest; so weak she can scarcely talk. Talking produces weakness in the arms. Nausea in the throat. Sensation of hollowness. Crowing, snorting respiration. Great sore feeling in the chest. Nape of neck weak. Feels as if she would faint. So weak on awaking, it puts her out of breath to dress. *Pains increase and decrease slowly.*

STRAMONIUM.

Labor:

Fainting spells, long continued, or frequent occurring. She suddenly falls with pale face and almost imperceptible breathing. Face bloated, red. Talks in an imploring and beseeching manner.

ABORTION.—Threatened *with unceasing loquacity;* she talks, prays, sings, constantly uttering something in this line; many hallucinations.

HÆMORRHAGE.—With delirium, *excessive loquacity, singing and praying.* Full of strange absurd ideas. Imagines she sees rats, mice, vermin, snakes, etc., and looks for them under the bed. Drawing pains in limbs and abdomen. Lifting the head frequently from the pillow, or starts up and looks around as if in fright. Abnormal sexual excitement. From retained placenta, with delirium. Discharge in large clots.

RETAINED PLACENTA.—With hæmorrhage and delirium.

CONVULSIONS.—*She appears terrified and shrinks back from every object on opening her eyes;* or she looks under the bed for vermin and *reptiles* which she fancies are there. Sardonic grinning. Stammering or loss of speech. Face red and puffed up. Loss of consciousness and sensibility. *Cries and frightful visions.* Laughter and singing, and efforts to escape. Copious perspiration with the spasms. Spasms are caused or renewed by brilliant objects, water, and sometimes by contact. Frightened appearance before and after the spasm commences. Abdomen puffed. Averse to water. *Continually lifting the head from the pillow.*

GENERALITIES.—The mania or delirium is of a wild character, the face being of a bright red; the eyes have a wild and suffused look, although not thoroughly congested. The hallucinations terrify her; she sees objects springing up from every corner; animals of every impossible kind arise to terrify her. Eyes open and pupils widely dilated. Decidedly loquacious. At times she may have a merry mood in her loquacity, and at others she has the horrors. At one moment she will be laughing, singing and making faces, and at another praying, crying for help, etc. Often has photomania; seems to have a perfect fear of the dark. May insist that she is conversing with spirits. At times she will be very silly; her talk is in a foolish and nonsensical manner and laughs at her own wit. The spasmodic motions are characterized by gracefulness rather than angularity; they are more gyratory than jerking. The tongue is red or whitish and covered with fine red dots, and is dry and parched; sometimes swollen and hangs out of the mouth. Nymphomania. Absence of pain is characteristic. *Can't bear* solitude or darkness. *Cannot walk* or keep on the feet in *a darkened room*, is sure to fall. While sleeping quietly the head is lifted from the pillow; or she starts up and looks around as in fright. The *first* sight of objects, persons,

etc., seem to alarm, stares in fright till she
finds there is no cause for fear. Eyes fixed
on dark side of room, away from the light.
Illusions of colors. Light dazzles. Face
red, bloated, hot; red, eyes wild; hot and
red, with cold hands and feet; pale. Difficult swallowing. Averse to fluids; shrinks
from the proffered cup. Averse to water,
even the sight of it causes spasms. Hydrophobia. The voice is higher and finer;
screeching; indistinct. Frequent twitchings; sudden jerks through the body. Hysteria. Arms agitated, lower limbs quiet.
Muscles will not obey the will.

SULPHUR.

Labor :

Pains ceasing. Pains too weak. Flushes
of heat; frequent weak faint spells; wants
more air and to be fanned. Cold feet, heat
on vertex. Hour-glass contractions.

ABORTION.—Frequent flushes of heat, cold
feet, heat on the top of the head. Weak,
fainting spells. Eruptions on face and elsewhere. Flowing and itching hæmorrhoids.
She sleeps badly. Faint and hungry at 11

A.M. Vomits her food. Intolerant of noise. A slight effort causes great fatigue.

HÆMORRHAGE.—Chronic; she seems almost well and then is worse again; so on for days. Weakness, fainting, flushes of heat. Heat on vertex. Cold feet. Gets hungry spells.

RETAINED PLACENTA.—Hour-glass contractions. Flushes of heat; wants to be fanned; faintness and weakness.

CONVULSIONS.—After the spasm has foolish happiness and pride, thinks herself possessed of beautiful things; even rags seem beautiful.

AFTER-PAINS.—Pains are located especially in the uterus. Pains from sacrum around pubes and down the thighs. Scanty lochia. Feels badly in abdomen. Flushes of heat. Weak and faint spells. Feet cold or very hot, especially soles. Talking fatigues and excites the pains. Bleeding, itching hæmorrhoids.

GENERALITIES. — Peevishness. Fantastic illusions; turns everything into beauty, even old rags and sticks. Happy dreams, wakes up singing. Psoric women: feels good to scratch. *Sudden and frequent flushes* of heat all over the body. Urine fœtid, with greasy-looking pellicle on it. Burning in vagina. Itching of vulva. Promotes expulsion of moles or blighted conceptions, and averts the predisposition to abort in future pregnancies. Talking fatigues and excites the pains. Suffocative fits; wants doors and windows open; wants to be fanned. Sensation as if the heart were enlarged. Pain in small of back. Spasmodic jerking in whole body. Great debility and trembling. Sensation of a mouse running up arms to back, before epileptic fits. Cramps in the lower extremities, with hot flushes and weak, faint spells. Burning in the soles of the feet. Cannot walk or sit erect. Always feels worse before a storm. Dim vision; halo around the light.

SULPHURICUM ACIDUM.

Labor :

HÆMORRHAGE.—Sensation of trembling all over without trembling, with *passive flow*. Discharge dark and thin.

AFTER-PAINS.—Great sense of general weakness, or a sense of trembling all over, without actual trembling.

GENERALITIES.—Hasty, quick and restless in her actions. General *sensation* of trembling; feels as if trembling from head to foot. Feels as if the white of an egg were dried on the face. Cold, relaxed feeling about the stomach, making her long for stimulants. Vomit and belching very sour. In bruises of soft parts after Arnica. Affections arising from general debility. Impatience. Feels that everything must be done in a great hurry. Brain feels loose in forehead. Labor-like pains in abdomen, extending to hips and back. Shortness of breath. Shooting through the heart. Knees and ankles weak. Aversion to water; it chills the stomach unless mixed with spirits. Exhaustion. Pains gradually come and cease suddenly.

THUJA.

Labor:

Pains ceasing. Pains too weak. Syphilitic troubles which hinder the proper contractility.

ABORTION.—At end of the third month, commencing with a scanty discharge of blood for five days, then more and more profuse.

GENERALITIES.—Warts on any part of the body with little necks, fig warts; long warts, same size all the way out. Venereal diseases. Fixed ideas; as if a strange person was at her side; as if made of glass; as if a living animal were in her abdomen; as if soul and body were separated. Hurried, with ill-humor. Feels as if she cannot exist any longer. Extreme scrupulousness. Music causes weeping and trembling of feet. Vertigo with eyes shut, ceasing when opening them. Illusions of sight. Teeth decay at roots, crown sound. Child moves too violently during pregnancy. Short of breath. Palpitation. Pulsations.

TRILLIUM PENDULUM.

ABORTION.—Delicate, anæmic women, subject to uterine displacements. Flow mostly bright red, more rarely dark and clotted. Hæmorrhage predominates. Discharge dark; *profuse; bright red.*

HÆMORRHAGE.—Active, of thick, dark, clotted blood after confinement or abortion; or bright-red flux. Great pros'ration resulting. *Women who habitually flood profusely after every parturition.* Gushing of bright-red at the least motion. Sinking in the stomach. Pain in the back. Legs cold. Feels as if bones were broken. Discharge profuse; dark clotted; *bright red; worse from motion;* foetid; bright, with clots.

GENERALITIES.—Displaced uterus with consequent menorrhagia; flow profuse. Menses come on after overexertion, too long ride, etc., profuse. When sacro-iliac synchondroses feel as if falling apart, wants to be bound tightly. Feels as if bones were broken. Crowding sensation in the veins like a tightening up of the parts, worse in those in the legs and ankles.

USTILAGO.

Labor:

Pains deficient. Os soft, pliable, dilatable.

ABORTION.—Hæmorrhage predominates. Passive, long-continued hæmorrhage after abortion, from retained secundines. Huge clots or large lumps of blood. Bearing-down pain in uterine region as if everything would come through, and profuse flow, either dark or bright, and almost always clotted. Uterus enlarged, cervix tumefied or dilated. From uterine congestion; from uterine inertia. Discharge black; coagulated; continuous, but not profuse; dark; offensive, or fœtid; bright-red gushes; passive; bright red; intermittent.

HÆMORRHAGE.—Chronic passive. Slow, persistent oozing of dark blood, with small black clots. Dark semi-fluid, but not watery blood. *Uterine inertia. Bright red, partly fluid and partly clotted.* Digital examination causes oozing of blood with small black coagula. Discharge active; continuous: passive; clotted; dark clots; *bright red.*

AFTER-PAINS. — Prolonged bearing-down pains, uterus feels as if drawn into a knot. Lochial discharge too profuse, partly fluid and partly clotted.

GENERALITIES. — Depression of spirits. Things whirl before the eyes. Twitching of eyes, they seem to revolve in circles and dart from object to object. Eyes feel hot on closing the lids. Sudden pallor. Constant aching, referred to the mouth of the womb. Displaced uterus. Burning pain in cardiac region.

VERATRUM ALBUM.

Labor :

Fainting from slightest exertion or motion. Cold sweat on forehead. Excessive weakness; is obliged to move very slowly; can hardly raise her hand as every motion seems to increase her debility. The pains exhaust her very much. Weak and almost imperceptible pulse. Thirst for icy-cold water.

ABORTION.—Threatened; pains, with cold sweat, nausea, vomiting. Where there has been exhausting diarrhœa.

CONVULSIONS.—Cold sweat on forehead, pallor, collapse; anæmic, or violent cerebral congestion with bluish bloated face. Delirium, wild shrieks and tearing of the clothes. Labor-pains exhaust her, fainting on least motion. After sudden violent emotions. Froth at mouth.

GENERALITIES.—Marked debility or exhaustion from functional or physical disturbances. *Cold sweat on forehead*, with many complaints. Haughtiness. Delirium. Respiration oppressed. Craves refreshing things, *and very cold*. Sexual desire too strong, particularly in childbed. Vomiting and diarrhœa. Countenance changed, unnatural.

Mania, with desire to tear and cut. Loquacity. Wants to kiss everybody. Impudent behavior in childbed. Cursing. Eyes turned upward, showing only whites; protruding; fixed, watery, sunken, lustreless. Face collapsed, pale, bluish; of leaden hue; red in bed, becomes pale rising; alternately pale and red. Dyspnœa. Violent palpitation, with fainting. Electric jerks in limbs. Cramps in calves. Hands and feet icy cold. Sudden sinking of strength.

VERATRUM VIRIDE.

Labor:

Rigid os uteri with threatening convulsions. Plethora, *pulse full, hard and quick.* Head and chest congested.

Convulsions.—Great activity of the arterial system (Pyrogen). Before, during or after labor, especially where mania remains after convulsions cease. *Furious delirium.* Emotional causes, or albuminuria. Full, hard, quick pulse is characteristic. Cold, clammy sweat. Profound cerebral congestion; between convulsions she remains unconscious and lies in a deep sleep, face red, eyes injected. Constant burning distress in cardiac region. Heart's action powerful. Violent convulsive twitchings.

GENERALITIES.—Depression of spirits. *Congestions.* Twitching contortion of eyes, rolling of eyeballs. Face cold, bluish ; paleness of the lips and around alæ nasi. Convulsive twitching of the facial muscles. Mouth drawn down at one corner. Vomiting. Labored breathing, must sit up. Heart's beat loud, strong, with arterial excitement. Faintness and blindness. Violent spasms, like galvanic shocks. Tingling and pricking in the skin.

VIBURNUM OPULUS.

Labor :

Pains spasmodic, crampy. False pains preceding or following real labor-pains. Cramps in the abdomen shooting down the legs. Spasmodic contractions of the os uteri. Violent pains and cramps in the legs, thighs and abdomen. *Painful labor*, where there has been a history of violent after-pains. False labor-pains during any month of pregnancy.

ABORTION. — Spasmodic pains shooting from the uterus into the legs. *Frequent and very early miscarriages*, the ovum is expelled at every monthly period, thus causing a seeming sterility. *Labor-like pains of an extraordinary severity.* Pains predominating. In the early weeks or months of pregnancy. Profuse hæmorrhage, in gushes. Pains begin in back, come around either side of the hypogastrium and culminate in intense squeezing, cramping and bearing down, going down into the thighs.

HÆMORRHAGE.—Profuse during abortion, in gushes.

AFTER-PAINS. — Violent spasmodic or cramp-like pains. Spasmodic contractions of the os. Pains radiating down the thighs. Induced by large clots. In hysterical, nervous women.

GENERALITIES. — Depressed. Heaviness over the eyes and in eyeballs, must, at times, look twice to be sure of seeing an object. Severe bearing down, drawing in anterior muscles of thighs; heavy aching in sacral region and over pubes; occasional sharp, shooting pains over ovaries; pains make her so nervous she cannot sit still. Tired, bruised pain in muscles of back, from point of scapula to wing of ilium on each side, better from firm pressure. Buzzing feeling in hands, as if they would burst. Stupid feeling, as if she could not tell where she was.

VIBURNUM PRUNIFOLIUM.

Labor:

ABORTION. — *False pains. Very painful, cramp-like, labor-like pains in the uterus, with terrible cramps in the legs and abdominal muscles,* accompanied by a gush of bright-red blood from the uterus. Excessive nervous, hysterical excitement, hysterical spasms and threatened miscarriage. Women who have a history of dysmenorrhœa. Palpitation of the heart. Pains so severe as to threaten to rupture the membranes and bring on miscarriage. During any month of pregnancy.

HÆMORRHAGE.—Profuse flooding, with violent pains (Hale).

AFTER-PAINS.

GENERALITIES.—Partial loss of speech; voice indistinct. Partial loss of consciousness. Vertigo. Aching in eyeballs. Throat and mouth very dry. Spasmodic *dysmenorrhœa.* Difficult, irregular breathing, weak and sighing. Pulse weak and irregular, with great prostration, weakness and dizziness.

VISCUM ALBUM.

Labor:

Tearing pains.

HÆMORRHAGE.—Passive.

RETAINED PLACENTA.—Retained or incarcerated placenta; metrorrhagia.

AFTER-PAINS.—Intermittent, in multiparæ.

GENERALITIES.—Dyspnœa; slow, stertorous breathing, with drowsiness. Inability for the patient to rest in a reclining position. Pulse small and weak. Cardiac weakness. *Tearing pains* in any part of the body. Giddiness. Feels very *queer*, as if she must fall down. A *glow* rising from the feet to the head; seems to be on fire. Face very pale. Sensation as of a large spider crawling on back of hand. Epileptic convulsions. Paralysis.

XANTHOXYLON.

Labor:

Spasmodic contractions of the os uteri, in sandy-haired women who have had dysmenorrhœa, ovarian troubles, headaches, amenorrhœa and chronic coughs.

AFTER-PAINS.—Dreadful distress and pain. Excruciatingly severe, continuous; pains extending down along the genito-crural nerves. Lochia profuse and offensive. Spare habit, nervous temperament and delicate organization seem more particularly to call for this remedy, but it may be used where indicated with confidence. Highly recommended by many.

GENERALITIES.—Nervous, frightened feeling. Depression and weakness. Bewildered feeling. Peppery taste in mouth, fauces and throat. Fluttering in stomach; sense of fulness or pressure in stomach. Tight feeling about chest. Desire to take a long breath. Weakness in lower limbs. Neuralgic, shooting pains in limbs. Pricking sensation; shocks as from electricity.

ZINCUM METALLICUM.

Labor:

ABORTION.—Fidgetiness and restlessness of the feet and legs. A tendency to abort.

CONVULSIONS.—Where eruptions have recently disappeared, especially old eruptions.

Muscular twitchings. Coma and convulsions from cerebral exhaustion. Loss of sensation over the whole of the body. Mania from mental excitement: Somnambulism. (Some recommend Zinc where Phosphorus has failed, being indicated.)

GENERALITIES. — Unconsciousness. Feet constantly moving, fidgety. Cannot keep still; must be in motion all the time. Thinks of death calmly. Pressure at root of nose. Eyes dim, watery. Pterygium. Face pale, alternately with redness. Sensation like a worm creeping up from pit of stomach to throat. Sudden oppression of the stomach. Pain in chest, as if cut to pieces. Feels as if a cap were over heart. Pulse irregular; scarcely perceptible. Sudden sensation of weakness in limbs, with canine hunger. Twitching in various muscles. The whole body jerks during sleep. Yawning. Complaints during absence of menses, *but feels perfectly well during the flow.* Better while eating.

PART II.

REPERTORIES.

PART II.

REPERTORIES.

LABOR.

ABDOMEN, bearing down, great, seems to be
only in the walls of, Agaric.

bloated, with, K. carb.

cramps in, with shooting down the legs,
Viburn. op.

cramps in, Gels.

cutting pains in, with, Phos., Puls.

cutting pains in, from before backward
and upward, with, Gels.

jerk-like tearing down the sides of, with,
Calc.

pains in, with, Cham.

pains, flying from side to side in, with,
Cimic.

prolonged urging in, with, Sec.

sensitive, very, across the, with, Con.

spasmodic, inefficient pains in various
parts of, with, Caul.

Abdomen, tenderness over the, with, Chlorof.
     weak feeling in, with, Phos., Sep.
Air, desire to have cool, fresh, with, Cham.,
         China, *Puls.*, Sec., Sulph.
     sensitive to currents of cool, with, Nux v.
Amniotic fluid gone, with, Bell.
Anguish, with, *Acon.*, Natr. c., Plat.
Ascend.   See Upward.
Answer, cannot give a civil, Cham.
Anus, sensation as of a weight in, as from a
         heavy ball, with, *Sep.*
Anxiety, with, Acon.
Appearing and disappearing suddenly of
         pains, *Bell.*, Magn. phos.
Back, bearing down from, to pelvis, with, K.
         carb.
     distressing, sore, aching pain in, with,
         Caust.
     drawing pains in, with, Nux v.
     drawing pains in, from back to thighs,
         with, Bell.
     feels as if it would break, with, Bell.
     great soreness of, with, Arn., Chlorof.
     Pains cutting across lumbar region,
         with, K. carb.
     pains in, descending thence to thighs,
         with, Nux v.

Back, pains in, violent, low down, Lob. i.
    pains going through to, and up the, with, Gels.
    pains lingering in, and passing down the buttocks, with, K. carb.
    pains start all right, then break and run up the, Gels.
    pains worse in, with, *Caust.*, Cocc., Coff., *Nux v.*, *Puls.*
    pressed, she wants her, K. carb.
    tearing pains begin in, radiating down the inner side of the legs, Cham.
Bear the pains, can hardly, Cham.
Bearing-down pains, as if contents of pelvis would be ejected, with Bell.
    down pains, great, seems to be only in the abdominal walls, Agaric.
Bed feels very hard to her, Bell.
    feels very hot to her, Op.
Belching, with relief from, K. carb., Mag. mur.
Bladder, constant pressure on, with, Lil. t.
    irritation of, with, Erig.
Breath, she is out of, Stann.
Breathing. See Respiration also.
    deeply with, Ign.
    difficult, with, *Acon.*, Ant. tart., Chin. s., Lob. i., *Puls.*, Sep.

Breathing, imperceptible, Stram.

    slow, through the mouth, Lyc.

Bruised feeling in the body, with, Arn.

      feeling of the abdominal walls and intestines, with, Nux v.

Burning in the parts, with, Calc.

Carotids, with throbbing, Bell.

Ceasing, pains, Acon., *Arn.*, BELL., Borax, Camph., Carb. v., Caul., *Cham.*, China, CIMIC., Cocc., Coff., Ign., Jab., K. CARB., Lyc., Mag. mur., *Natr. mur.*, *Nux v.*, OP., PULS., *Ruta*, SEC., *Sep.*, Sulph., Thuj.

Cervix uteri, with needle-like pains in, Caul.

    induration of, Sep.

      with shooting pains in, extending upward, Sep.

      soft, flabby, no attempt at expulsion, Gels.

      stinging, stitches in the, Calc.

      thick, leathery, *Lob. i.*

Cessation of pains (entire), Acon., Carb. v., *Cimic.*, Cinnam., *Gels.*, Graph., (Guar.), *Nux v.*

    from hæmorrhage, China, Cimic., Puls.

    sudden, and coma sets in between convulsive paroxysms, Op.

Cheeks, one red, the other pale, Cham.
  fiery red, Fer.
Chest, congestion of, with, Aur., Nux v.,
      Verat. v.
    pains go up to, Gels.
    sensation of fulness in, with, Cactus.
    sensation of weakness in, with, Stann.
Chilliness, with, Ars., Cimic., Nux m., Puls.
Chills, nervous, in first stage, with, Gels.
Coldness of the body, with, Camph., China.
    of the extremities, with, Sep.
Cold, the least, almost unendurable, Calc.
Complains that she cannot bear the pains,
      Acon.
    that the child "lies so queer," Puls.
Constriction around the pelvis, painful, ex-
      tending gradually towards the stom-
      ach, Cactus.
Constrictive pains in the first stage, imped-
      ing dilatation of the os, Nux v.
Contracted, parts feel, Acon.
Contractions, hour-glass. See Hour-glass
      Contractions.
    prevented by syphilitic troubles, Thuj.
    severe, of the fundus, with constriction
      of the os, Caul.
Contractive pains in the left side of the
      uterus, with, Puls.

Convulsions. See Repertory on Convulsions.

    with, China, Chlorof., Cinnam., Op., Sec.

    hysterical interrupt, Magn. m.

    threatened, Verat. v.

Cool, with body, Arn.

Covered, desire to be, with, Ars., Sep.

    will not be, during, Camph., Sec.

Cramps in abdomen, shooting down the legs, with, Viburn. op.

    with, Cimic.

    in lower extremities, with, Cupr.

    in the uterine region, with, Plat.

Crazy, declares she will go, Cimic.

    feels as if she will go, Coff.

Cutting pains, with, Gels., Ip.

    pains in the abdomen, with, Phos.

    pains in the abdomen, from before, backward and upward, with, Gels.

    pains low down in abdomen, with sensation as if stool would occur, Puls.

    pains from hip to foot, worse from touch or motion, with, Bry.

    in the hypogastrium, with, Calc.

    dragging in the hypogastrium, extending around the loins, with, Puls.

Darting pains, with, Ip.

Death, with extreme fear of, Acon., Coff.

Debility, with, *Ars.*, Carbo. v., Caust., *Fer.*,
     Iod., *K. carb.*, Lyc., Lob. i., *Mur. ac.*,
     Nux v., Sep., Verat. a.

  after labor, with, Caust.

  consult, also, Exhaustion.

Deficient pains, with. See Weak pains, too.

Delirium, with, Hyosc.

Desperate, pains make her, Aur.

Digging pains, with, China.

Distension of veins of head and neck, with,
     Chin. s.

Distress, with, great, Acon., Amyl. nit., Arn.,
     Aur., Bell., Puls.

Distressing pains, with, Arn., CHAM., Cimic.,
     Coff., Con., GELS., K. CARB., Lyc.,
     Nux v., Phos., Puls., *Sec.*, SEP.

Downward motion, she fears a, Borax.

  pressure, with desire for stool or urine,
     Nux v.

Dragging in the groins, with, Calc.

Drawing pains, from small of back to thighs,
     with, Bell.

  pains from hip to foot, with, Bry.

  pains in the uterine ligaments, with,
     Caul.

  pressive pains, extending toward the
     uterus, with, Puls.

Dreads beforehand the approaching confinement, Gels.

Drowsiness.   See Sleepiness.

Dryness of the parts, with, Acon.

    also see the various parts.

Dyspnœa. See Breathing, difficult.

Ears, ringing in (noises), China.

Endure the pains, she cannot, Cham.

Eructations violent, with, Borax.

    with many, Carb. v.

    with relief from, K. carb., Mag. mur.

Examination, intolerant of, from local sensitiveness, Acon., Arn., *Plat.*

    intolerant of, from nervousness, Bell., China, Gels.

    will not permit, snappish, Cham.

Excitement, nervous, with, Cham., *Cimic.*, *Coff.*, Morph. ace.

Exhaustion, with, *Ars.*, Caul., *China*, Con., Iod., *K. carb.*, Lyc., Rhus t., Stram., Sulph.

    from long protracted labor, Caul.

    in leuco-phlegmatic women, Calc.

    pains seem to cause, and to make speech difficult, Stann.

    consult, also, Debility.

Exhausts her, pains, Verat. a.

Eyes, convulsive motion of muscles of, Chin.
      s., Hyosc.
    half open, with, Lyc.
    injected with, Bell., Op.
Face bloated, with, Ars., Op., Stram.
    bluish color of, with, Hyosc.
    convulsive action of muscles of, with,
        Chin. s., Hyosc.
    dark red, with, Op.
    flushed up, with, *Arn.*, (Amm. c.), Amyl
        nit., *Bell.*, Fer., Gels.
    flushed, dark, with, Gels.
    hot, with, Bell.
    pale, with, Ars., Fer., Hyosc., Nux m.,
        Puls., Stram.
Fainting, with, *Acon.*, Arn., *Ars.*, Bell., Bry.,
        Camph., Carb. v., *Cham.*, *China*,
        Cimic., Cinnam., Cocc., *Coff.*, Dig.,
        Ign., Ip., Lach., Mag. mur., Nux m.,
        Nux v., Puls., Rhus t., Sec., *Sep.*,
        Stram., Sulph., Verat. a.
    from least motion, Bry.
    from sensitiveness to pain, Cham.
    long continued and frequent, Stram.
False pains, Arn., *Bell.*, Borax, CAUL., *Cham.*,
        Cimic., Cinnam., *Coff.*, Gels., K. carb.,
        K. phos., *Nux m.*, *Nux v.*, *Puls.*, Sec.,
        Sep., Viburn. op., *Viburn. pr.*

False pains, with bloody discharge, Sec.

Fanned, desire to be, Carb. v., China, Puls., Sulph.

Fatigue, every exertion produces, Calc. see Debility.

Fear, with, *Acon.*, Ars. that she will die, *Acon.*, Coff., Plat. that something will certainly go wrong, Acon.

Feeble pains. See Weak Pains.

Feet, cold, damp, clammy, Calc.

Fever, with, Caul.

Fingers, with cramps in, Cupr.

Flatulency, with, Lyc. after labor, Nux m.

Foot against a support, and pressing and relaxing alternately, relief by, Lyc.

Forcing pains, with Mag. phos., *Sec.*

Forebodings, with, Natr. m.

Frantic, pains make her, Cham.

Frequent pains, with, Acon.

Fright, pains ceasing from, Acon.

Get up, says she will and must, Cham.

Grief, with, Caust., Ign.

Griping in the hypogastrium, with, Calc. pains in the uterus, with, Cham.

Hands touched, cannot bear to have, during, China.

Hard pain, followed by several light ones,
  Cocc.

Hæmorrhage, with, *Bell.*, Cham., China,
  Cinnam., Erig., Fer., Hyosc., *Ip.*,
  Lyc., Plat., *Sabi.*, *Sec.*

  see under Repertory on Hæmorrhage.

Head, congestion to, with, Arn., Aur., Nux
  v., Verat. v.

  heat on the vertex, with, Sulph.

  hot, with cool body, Arn.

Headache, with, Acon., Amyl. nit., Bell.,
  Cham., Cimic., Cocc., Gels., Glon.,
  Hyosc., Nux v.

  throbbing with, Bell., Cocc.

Hearing, with dull, Cham.

Heart, palpitation of, with, Aur., *Puls.*

Heat, flushes of, with, Sep., Sulph.

Help, calls for, Cham.

Hips, cramps in, during, Cimic.

  numb, paralyzed feeling in, during,
    Cocc.

  pains extend to the, Gels.

  twitching, tearing in the, Mag. mur.

  uterine spasms extending to the, Mag.
    mur.

Hollow, whole body feels, as if empty, K.
  carb.

Hot parts, with, Acon., Bell.

Hour-glass contractions, *Bell.*, *Cham.*, Cocc., Con., Cupr., Hyosc., *K. carb.*, Nux v., *Plat.*, Puls., Rhus t., *Sec.*, *Sep.*, Sulph.

Hysteria, with, Ign., Mag. mur.

Impatience, with, Cham.

Ineffectual pains, with, Acon., Arn., Cimic., Cinnam., Coff., Gels., Goss., K. carb., K. phos., Phos., Plat., Puls., Sec.
    see also, weak, pains too.

Inertia, uterine, Caust., China, Gels., PULS., Sec.

Insupportable pains, with, Acon.

Intermitting pains, with, CAUL.

Interrupted pains, by sensitiveness of the vagina and parts, *Plat.*

Irregular pains, with, Arn., Aur., Caul., Caust., Cocc., Cupr., Nux m., Nux v., Puls., Sec.

Irritability, with, Cham., Hyosc., Nux v.

Jarring of the bed, sensitive to, Bell.

Jerking, with, Op.
   — see Twitching.

Lamenting, with, Cham., Cimic., Coff., Lyc.

Lancinating pains. See Cutting Pains.

Left side, pains all on the, Plat.

Left to right, pains go from, Ip.

Legs, cramping in the, with, Cupr., Mag. phos.

    each pain attended by sudden sharp cramps in calves of, Nux v.

    heavy and torpid, with, Cimic.

    numb and paralyzed feeling in, with, Cocc.

    pains shooting down the, with, Viburn. op.

    pains tearing down the, with, Cham.

Lie down, desire to, Fer.

Light, sensitive to the, with, Bell., Con.

Lingering, almost painless labor, Goss.

    pains, see Slow Pains.

Located, pains not rightly, *Cimic.*

    child not rightly, feels as if, *Puls.*

Loins, pains in, cause constant urging to stool, Nux v.

Maids, especially in old, muscles rigid, Bell.

Melancholy, with, Cimic., Ign., Lach., Natr. m., Puls.

Moaning, with, Acon., Bell., Cham.

Motion, all her motions are quick, Bell.

    choreic, all over, with, Cimic.

    fears a downward, she, Borax.

    must keep in constant, Lyc.

Motion, of the child, painful, Arn., Puls.
    worse from, Bry.
Moving about, better when, Nux m.
Nausea, with, *Ant. tart.*, Caul., Cham., *Cocc.*,
    IP., Mag. mur., *Puls.*
Near, cannot bear any one, Cham.
Needle-like pains, with, Sep.
Nervousness, with, Cham., Cimic., Gels.,
    Iod., Nux v.
Neuralgic pains in uterus, with, Cimic.,
    Lil. t.
Noise, sensitive to, Bell., Cimic., Borax.
Numb feeling, with, Caust., Cocc.
Open and loose without action, everything
    seems, Sec.
Os uteri, contracted with throat and heart
    symptoms, Lach.
    dilated, but patient has become tired
        and fretful, with, Caust.
    dilatable, soft, with deficient pains, Ustil.
    dilatation impeded by constrictive
        pains in first stage, Nux v.
    dry, with, Acon.
    hot, with, Bell.
    irregularly constricted, now dilatable,
        now suddenly closed by spasm,
        Cimic.

Os uteri, rigidity of, *Ant. tart.*, Bell., CAUL., *Cham.*, Chlorof., *Cimic.*, GELS., Ign., Jab., *Lob. i.*, Lyc., *Nux v.*, Sec., VERAT. V.

    spasmodic contractions of, *Acon.*, Amyl. nit., BELL., Cactus., CAUL., CIMIC., Con., Hyosc., Lach., Lyc., Morph. ace., Sec., *Viburn. op.*, Xan.

    stinging, stitches, in the, Calc., Con.

    tender, with, Bell.

    tender and undilatable, with, Acon.

    thick, with, Gels., Lob. i.

    thin, with, Bell.

Ovaries, pains in, extending down inside of thighs, with, Lil. t.

Painful labor, extremely, Cham., Plat..

    labor, with previous history of violent after-pains, Viburn. op.

Palpitation. See Heart, Palpitation of.

Paralysis of sphincter vesicæ, after, Chlorof.

Paralytic pains, with, Cocc.

Peevishness, with, Cham.

Perinæum, rigidity of, Lob. i.

Perspiration, with, Natr. c., Puls.

    cold, clammy, with, Dig., Hyosc.

    cold on forehead, with, Verat. a.

    head and upper part of body, about the, Calc.

Perspiration, hot, with, Acon.

Placenta descends with the head, Cinnam.

Position, must change, often, Arn., Rhus t.
   complains that the child is in the
      wrong, Puls.

Presentation, abnormal, *Puls.*

Primiparæ, especially suited to the, Bell.

Progress, slow, with, Bell., Caul., Chlorof.,
   Goss., Ign., Natr. m., Puls., Stann.

Prolapsus uteri, after labor, Ruta.

Prolonged pains, with, Sec.

Prostration.   See Exhaustion.

Pulsations in arteries with, Iod., K. carb.

Pulse, full, hard, quick, with, Verat. v.
   intermitting, with, Chin. s., Dig., K. phos.
   loss of, or nearly so, with, China.
   rapid, with, Chin. s.
   very slow, irregular, with, Dig.
   weak, with, Camph., K. phos., Sec.,
      Verat. a.

Rapid succession, pains in, Acon.

Rectum, constant pressure on the, with,
   Lil. t.
   irritation of, with, Erig.

Relaxed, everything seems, during, Caust.,
   Sec.

Respiration, sighing, with, Bry.
   see Breathing.

Restlessness, with, ACON., Arn., ARS., Camph., *Cham.*, Chlorof., *Cimic.*, K. carb., Nux m., *Rhus t.*

    between the pains, especially, Cupr.

Right to left, pains go from, Lyc.

Rigid, parts feel, with, Acon.

    os. See under Os Uteri and also Vagina.

Rubbed, desire to be, which relieves, during, Natr. c.

Sacrum, bearing down in region of, with, Sec.

    drawing from, forward, with. Cham.

    pains from, direct through to pubes, with, Sabi.

    pains in, after labor, Phos.

    pains in, distressing, Lob. i.

    with only slight pressure on, instead of regular pains, with, Bell.

Sadness. See Melancholy.

Sensitiveness to pain, great. See Distressing Pains.

    after labor, she cannot bear the touch even of the napkin, Plat.

    to external impressions, odors, etc. Nux v.

Severe pains, with, CHAM., Cimic., *Coff.*, Con., Morph. ace., Puls., *Sec.*, SEP.

    see also Violent Pains.

Sharp pains, with, K. carb.

Shivers (in first part of labor) with the pains, Cimic.

Shooting pains through whole body, Lob. i.

Short pains, with, Caul.

Shrinks from the pains, Cham.

Shuddering during, wants to be covered, Sep.

Sighing, with, Ign., Lob. i.

Similar, pains, Camph., Cham., Kreo.

Skin cold, with, Camph., Sec.

    cool, dry, no sweat, Nux m.

Sleepiness (drowsy), with, Gels., Nux m., Op.

Sleeplessness, with, Con., Mag. mur.

Slow pains, with, Bell., Con., Cimic., Gels., Hyperc., Nux m., Puls., Sec.

    labor, Bell., Goss., Jab., K. phos., Natr. m., Nux v., Puls., Stann.

Sobbing, with.   See Weeping.

Sopor, with, Op.

Soreness all over, with, *Arn.*, Ruta.

    apparently resulting from abnormal sensitiveness of the cervix to the pressure of the child's head, Arn.

    in the parts, Calc.

    of the uterus and abdominal walls, with, Puls.

Spasms, labor-pains appear like tonic, Chin. s.

  uterine, extending to the hips, with, Mag. mur.

Spasmodic pains, Amyl. nit., *Bell.*, Borax, CAUL., Caust., CHAM., *Cimic.*, *Cocc.*, Con., Cupr., Fer., GELS., HYOSC., *Ip.*, Lyc., Mag. phos., Nux m., *Nux v.*, Plat., PULS., *Sec.*, *Sep.*, Stann., Viburn. op.

  see, also, under Os Uteri.

  pains flying about, but *not* in normal direction, Caul.

Spitefulness, with, Cham.

Stitching pains, with, K. carb.

Stomach, distressed, empty feeling in pit of, Sep.

  pains more violent in, than in uterus, Borax.

  spasmodic pains in the, Caul.

Stool, with urging to, Lil. t., Nux v.

  with retention of, Op.

Strong pains, too. See Severe.

Stupid, she is, Gels.

Sudden pains, with, Bell.

Suicide, tempted, Aur.

Suppression of pains, with, Nux m., Sec.

Suppression of pains from fear, Op.

    of pains from fright, Op.

    see, also, Ceasing, Pains.

Suspiciousness, with, Cimic.

Sweat. See Perspiration.

Talks imploringly, Stram.

    nonsensical, yet she seems conscious of what she is doing, but says she cannot help it, Cimic.

    chattering, during first stage, Gels.

Tardy pains. See Slow Pains.

    labor. See Slow Labor.

Tearing pains, with, CHAM., China, *Cimic.*, *Visc. alb.*

Tedious labor. See Slow Labor.

    pains. See Slow Pains.

Tenderness of the parts, with, Acon., Bell., Plat.

Terror, mental, with, Cocc.

Thick, leathery cervix, *Lob. i.*

Thighs, aching in the, with, Calc.

    drawing pains in the, with, Nux v.

    violent pains and cramps in the, with, Viburn. op.

Thirst, with, Ars., Caul., Cham., K. carb.

    for cold water in large quantities, Bry.

    for icy-cold water, Verat. a.

Thirstlessness, with, Puls.

Thoughts, her, horrify her, Plat.

Toes, cramps in, Cupr.

Tormenting, useless, pains in the beginning of labor, with, Caul.

Touch, sensitive to, especially about the throat, Lach.

Touched, during, cannot bear to be, China.

Trembling, with, Cocc., Fer., Gels., Ign., Nux v.

Tremor, with, Fer., Natr. c.

Twitching, with, Chin. s., Cimic., Cinnam., Hyosc., Op.

Umbilicus, sharp cutting pains about, which dart off toward the uterus, *Ip.*

Unconsciousness, after labor, Chin. s.

Undilatable parts, with, ACON.
    look to the cause.

Upward, pains go, Borax., Lyc.
    pains force child, Borax., Cham., Gels.
    uterus seems to go, Cimic.

Urinate, with urging to, Lil. t., Nux v.
    inability to, from paralytic condition of bladder, Caust.

Urine, with retention of, Op., Lyc.
    frequent emissions of large quantities of pale, *Cham.*
    red sand in, Lyc.

Useless, tormenting pains in the beginning of labor, Caul.

Uterus, fatigue of the, ARN.

    inertia of. See Inertia.

    see, also, Os Uteri.

Vagina, dry, with, Acon., Bell., Fer., Jab.

    hot, with, Acon., Bell., Jab.

    more or less discharge of dark coagulated blood from, Cham.

    profuse secretion of mucus from, Caul.

    rigidity of, with, Ars.

    sensitiveness of, interrupting labor pains, Plat.

    tender and undilatable, with, Acon.

    too small, can hardly introduce the finger, Ars.

Vertigo, with, Cham., China.

    on turning in bed, with, Con.

Violent pains, with, Acon., Arn., *Bell.*, *Nux v.*

    pains, but do little good, Arn., Caul., Coff., Phos., Plat.

    see, also, Severe Pains.

Vision, with dim, Cham., Cimic.

    of rats, etc., Cimic.

Vomiting, with, Cocc.

    consult Nausea.

Vulva, dry, with, Acon.

Vulva, rigidity of the, with, Coff.
>> tender and undilatable, with, Acon.
>> varicose condition of the, Carb. v.

Walk about for relief, pains make her, Puls.

Wave, sensation of, from uterus to throat,
>> which seems to impede labor, Gels.

Weak pains, too, Arn., BELL., Borax,
>> Camph., Carb. v., *Caul.*, *Caust.*, *Cham.*,
>> China, CIMIC., Cinnam., Cocc.,
>> GELS., Goss., Graph., Ign., K.
>> CARB., K. phos., Lyc., Mag. mur.,
>> Natr. c., *Natr. m.*, Nux m., *Nux v.*,
>> OP., Plat., PULS., *Ruta*, SEC., *Sep.*,
>> Sulph., Thuj., Ustii., Zinc.
>> patient too, to develop normal pains,
>> Caul., Mur. ac.

Weakness, muscular, Gels.
>> see Debility.

Weariness, sense of, with, Arn.

Weeping, with, Coff., Lyc., Lob. i., Ign., Plat.
>> Puls.

Window, desire to jump out of the, Aur.
>> open, desire to have, Puls.

Women, corpulent, in, Graph.
>> cachectic, in, Sec.
>> blondes, in, Viburn. op.
>> tall, slender, in, Phos.

Wrapped up, desire to be. See Covered, desire to be.

ABORTION.

(Consult, also, Repertories on Labor and Hæmorrhage.)

ABDOMEN, bearing down, great, seems to be in the walls of, Agaric.

> contraction around the hypochondria, painful, Rhus. t.

> contractive pain in, with terrible bearing down, Sep.

> cramps in the muscles of, Viburn. op.

> drawing from, to the backbone, as if by a string, Plb.

> fainting and sinking in the, feeling of, Sabi.

> fermentation, in constant state of, with pains shooting from right to left, Lyc.

> heaviness in, with, Cham., Sep.

> labor-like pains in, alternating with hæmorrhage, Puls.

> pains in, extending to the sides, Cham.

> pains fly across from side to side, especially right to left, Cimic.

> pains in, sharp, distressing, run upward, or upward and backward, Gels.

Abdomen, pains in, shoot across from right to left, Lyc.

    sensation as if tight, would break with much effort to void stool, Apis.

    sensation of something alive in the, Croc.

    sensation of distension of, or as if bloated, as if packed full. Chin.

    soft and relaxed, Sabi.

    soreness, much, in, Ham.

    spasms in, with, Carb. v., Nux v.

    stitching pains in, K. carb.

Abortion, cause of. See the various causes.

Aching, violent, and tensive pains through whole body, with sensation of constriction and tension, Bell.

Afraid to turn over, to move, or to leave the bed, Acon.

After-birth, retention of, *Bell.*, *Canth.*, *Caul.*, Cimic., Gels., Goss., *Puls.*, *Sabi.*, *Sec.*, Sep., Visc. alb.

    retention of. See, also, Repertory on Retained Placenta.

Agony, great, referred to the uterine region, Cham.

Air, wants fresh, Puls.

Anæmia, from, *Alet. far.*, Calc., China, Fer.,

Helon., K. carb., Plb., Puls., Sec., Trill.

Anger, from, Acon., Cham.

Anus, prolapsus of, with stool, Pod.

sense of weight in, like a heavy ball, *Sep.*

Anxiety, with great nervous excitability, *Acon.*

Appetite, loss of, Sulph.

Back, contracting, out-pressing pain from, to front, worse lying in bed, Cham.

pain in, as if it would break, *Bell.*, *K. carb.*

pain in, coming around either side of the hypogastrium and culminating in intense squeezing, Viburn. op.

pain in, drawing, Rhus t.

pain in, extending through to pubes, Sabi.

pain in, extending into thighs, Cimic., K. carb., Viburn. op.

pain in, intolerable before urinating, with almost entire relief with the flow, Lyc.

pain in, paralytic, legs almost useless, Cocc.

pain in renal region, stitching in the, K. carb.

Back, pain in, severe, and in loins, Caul.
 pain in small of, Asar., Bell., Calc., Lyc.
 pain in small of, with great weakness,
  K. carb.
 pain in, when walking, K. carb.
 pain in, when walking feels that she
  must sit down, K. carb.
 pain in, worse from motion, Bry.
 weak, with, K. carb.
Bearing down pains, with, *Bell.*
 down pains, great, seem to be in the abdominal walls only, Agaric.
 down pains, spasmodic, Caul.
Bed, afraid to leave the, Acon.
 feels too hard, Arn.
 feels too hot, Op.
 worse lying in the, Cham.
 vertigo when turning over in, Con.
Belching, with relief, Arg. nit.
Blindness, momentary attacks of, in a warm
  room, Sep.
Blood poisoning, from, Crotal., *Pyrog.*
Breathless, or almost so, China.
Bruise, from a, Arn.
Bruised, she feels, *Arn.*
Catarrh, disposition to, Camph., Sep., Sulph.
Cellar, from living in cold, damp, Dulc.

Cervix uteri, fine darting pains in, Sep.

    hard lumps on, Kreo.

    induration of, from, Aur., Con., Sep.

    tumefied or dilated, Ustil.

Chest, congestion to the, Sep.

    fulness and pressure in the, Sep.

    trembling sensation in middle of the, Rhus t.

    weak feeling in the, Stann.

Child feels as if it laid crosswise, Arn.

    motion of, excessive, Lyc.

    motion of, painful, Arn.

    very feeble, scarcely perceptible, Sep.

Chilliness, with, Cham., Nux m., Puls.

Chills, nervous, Gels.

    for several days, with pricking in the chest, Cimic.

Cold or damp, from, Acon., Dulc., Puls., Rhus t.

Coldness of the body, with, Camph., Dig.

Colic, with, Calc., Sep.

Concussions, shocks, falls, from, *Arn.*, Cinnam., Con., *Rhus i.*

    especially if she begins to flow with or without pain, or pain with or without flow, Arn.

Congestion, from uterine, Alet. far., Bell.,

Canth., Caul., China, Cimic., Croc., (Hep.), Nux v., Sep., Ustil.

Congestion, from passive uterine, Caul., Sec., Ustil.

from uterine with ulceration, Canth.

Constipation, with, Apis., Bry., (Collin.), K. carb., Nux v., Op., Phos., Plb., Sep., Sil.

Constriction, sense of, in body, with Bell.

Contracting, out-pressing pains from back to front, worse lying in bed, Cham.

Contractions, uterine, feeble, tormenting, irregular, and with very slight hæmorrhage, Caul.

Convulsions, with, Cimic., Hyosc., Ip., Plat., Sec.

consult Repertory on Convulsions.

of the limbs, with restlessness, Cham.

Convulsive movements, Sec.

Cramps in calves of the legs, Rhus t.

Cystitis, from, Acon., Cann. sat., Canth.

Damp or cold, from, Acon., Dulc., Puls., Rhus t.

or cold places, from, Dulc.

Death, fear of, with, Acon., Sec.

Debility. See Prostration.

Delirium, with, Hyosc.

Depression, mental, with, Nitr. ac., Plb.

Diarrhœa, with, Erig., Gels., Sabi., Verat. a.

Discharge. For quantity and character of the flow, see under Hæmorrhage, in this Repertory. Also consult Repertory on Hæmorrhage.

black, Asar., Cham., Croc., Kreo., Plat., Puls., Sec., Ustil.

black and coagulated, Cham., China, Croc., Puls., Sabi., Ustil.

black, thin and with foul-smelling clots, Sec.

black and stringy, Croc.

black in gushes, Puls.

black and thick, Plat.

black and offensive, Cham., Croc , Kreo., Sec.

bright red, Arn., *Bell.*, Cham., China, *Cinnam.*, Erig., Ham., *Hyosc.*, *Ip.*, Lac. c., *Millif.*, Puls., *Pyrog.*, *Sabi.*, Sec., Rhus t., *Trill.*, Ustil., Viburn. pr.

bright red, continuous, Hyosc., Ip.

bright red, not coagulating, Ham.

bright red, coagulating and with clots, Arn., Bell., Ip., Sabi., Ustil.

bright red, with dark clots, Pyrog.

clots, foul smelling, Sec.

Discharge, clots or stringy masses form as
　　　rapidly as it flows from vulva, Croc.

　　coagulated, Arn., Bell., Cham., China,
　　　Croc., Fer., Helon., Ip., Kreo., Plat.,
　　　Puls., Sabi., Sec., Trill., Ustil.

　　dark, Bell., Bry., Canth., Cham., China,
　　　Croc., Crotal., Fer., Helon., Kreo.,
　　　Nux m., Plat., Puls., Sabi., Sec.,
　　　Trill., Ustil.

　　dark and coagulated, Bell., Cham., China,
　　　Croc., Fer., Puls., Sabi., Sec., Ustil.

　　dark fluid, Bry., Crotal., Plat., Sabi.,
　　　Sec.

　　dark and offensive, Bell., Cham., Croc.,
　　　Crotal., Kreo., Sabi., Sec., Ustil.

　　dark and thick, Nux m., Plat.

　　corroding, Kreo.

　　hot, *Bell.*, Lac. can.

　　lumpy.　See Coagulated.

　　partly bright, partly composed of black
　　　strings, Croc.

　　serous mucus, Arn.

　　watery, China, Fer., Kreo., Sabi., Sec.

　　watery, with clots, China, Fer., Sabi.,
　　　Sec.

Disease, in the course of septic or zymotic,
　　　Crotal., Pyrog.

Dizziness, with, Acon.

Dreads abortion greatly, Nux m.

Drugs, or narcotics, from, Bell., (Hepar.),
        Nux v.

Dyspepsia, with, Alet. far., Nux v.

Early months, in the, Apis., Viburn. op.

Ears, ringing in the, China.

Emotions, sudden, depressing, from, Gels.
        irritating, from, Helon.

Eruptions on face and elsewhere, Sulph.

Excitability, with great nervous, Arn., *Acon.*,
        Cham., *Coff.*, Fer., Viburn. pr.

Excitement, with great vascular, Caul.

Exertion, over, from, Cinnam., Helon., Mil-
        lef., Nitr. ac., *Rhus t.*

Extremities, rigidity of the, Hyosc.
        followed by tearing pains in the, Sec.
        consult, also, Legs.

Eyes, red, with, *Bell.*
        with sacculated swelling over the, K.
            carb.

Face, bright-red, with, Fer.
        eruptions on the, with, Sulph.
        flushed, with red eyes, etc., Bell.
        paleness of, with exhaustion, Fer.
        pallor of, with, K. carb.
        yellow spots on the, Sep.

Faintness, with, Croc., Dig., Lyc., Nux m., Sep., Sulph.

Fall, from. See Concussion.

False labor pains. See Repertory on Labor.

Fear, with, Acon.

> great, of abortion occurring, Nux m.
>
> that something terrible will happen to her, Acon.
>
> see, also, Afraid.

Feet, cold, Sulph.

> cold, damp, Calc.
>
> fidgetiness of the, Zinc.

Fever, typhoid, from (Bapt.), (Pyrog.).

Fifth month to the seventh, Sep.

Fingers spread apart, she holds her, which worries her much, Sec.

First month, in, Croc., Viburn. op.

> half of pregnancy, during, Nitr. ac.

Flatus, desire to pass, without relief, China.

Flushes of heat, with faintness, and sense of blindness in warm room, Sep.

> of heat, cold feet, heat in vertex, Sulph.

Fœtus. See Child.

Fourth month, in, Apis.

Fright, from, *Acon.*, Cimic., Gels., *Op.*

Genitals, atony of the, with, Fer.

> swelling of the external, Merc.

Genitals, tender to touch, Sil.
   varices of the, Calc., *Carbo. v.*
   see, also, Vulva, Uterus, etc.
Glands, inguinal, swelling of the, Merc.
Gonorrhœa, from, Cann. sat.
Grief, suppressed, from, *Ign.*
Hæmorrhage. For Color and Character of
   the blood, see Discharge. Also
   consult Repertory on Hæmorrhage.
  after abortion (especially), China., Erig.,
   Ham., Millef., Nux m., Sil., Trill.
  arrested for a little while, then reappears with redoubled violence, Puls.
  bad effects of, China.
  bad effects of, at the third month,
   Kreo.
  comes and goes suddenly, Bell.
  coming on suddenly, Bell., Cinnam.
  continuous, Arn., Cinnam., Ham.,
   Hyosc., Ip., Sabi., Ustil.
  continuous bright-red, Hyosc., *Ip.*
  continuous, but not profuse, Ustil.
  continuous with nausea, Ip.
  continuous, obstinate, Nux m., Ustil.
  face, with fiery-red, Fer.
  false labor-pains, with, Sec.
  forerunner, as a, Ruta.

Hæmorrhage, genitals, external, with swelling of, and inguinal glands, Merc.

gushes in, Cham., China, Puls., Sabi., Sec., Ustil., Viburn. op.

Intermitting, Bell., China, Kreo., Puls., Rhus t., Sabi., Ustil.

motion, worse from, *Bry.*, Coff., Croc., Erig., *Sabi.*, Sec.

nausea, with, *Ip.*

oozing of dark blood, with small coagula for days, Ustil.

pain and, alternate, Puls.

pain, without, Arn., Sabi., Sec.

paroxysmal, Apocyn. c.

paroxysmal, brought on from the slightest motion, Sabi.

passive, Alet. far., Caul., China, *Croc.*, *Ham.*, Helon., *Sec.*, Ustil.

predominating (especially), Acon., Bell., China, Cinnam., Croc., Erig., Ham., Ip., Kreo. Millif., Nux m., Sabi., Sec., Trill., Ustil.

profuse, Apis, Arn., Bell., Cham., China, Cinnam., Croc., Erig., Fer., Helon., Hyosc., Ip., Millif., Sabi., Sec., Trill., Ustil., Viburn. op.

retained secundines, from, Goss., Ustil.

Hæmorrhage, scanty, Caul., Nux v., Thuj., Ustil.

  tendency to, Calc.

Habitual tendency to (Abortion), *Alet. far.*, Arg. nit., Asar., *Bapt.*, Calc., Cann. sat., Carb. v., Caul., Cimic., Cocc., Fer., Helon., *K. carb.*, Kreo., Lyc., Nux m., Plb., Puls., Ruta, *Sabi.*, *Sep.*, Sil., Sulph., Viburn. op., Zinc.

  always at the same time, usually caused by some induration of uterus, Aur.

  from non-development of the uterus, Plb.

  usually too profuse and too early menses, Calc.

Hæmorrhoids, flowing and itching, with, Sulph.

Hallucinations, with many, Stram.

Head, aching of the, Bry., Carb. v.

  confusion of, with, Arg. nit.

  confused feeling in, affecting the mind, Gels.

  congestion to, with, *Bell.*, Bry., *Calc.*, Sep., *Sulph.*

  congestion, frequent, with, Carb. v., Lyc.

  dulness, with, Arg. nit.

Head, heaviness of, with, China.
>> pain in, with, Arg. nit., Sep.
>> pain in, as if head would split, Bry.
>> perspiration about the, hot, with, China.
>> perspiration about the, cold, with, Verat. a.
>> pulsating, burning pain in, Phos.

Hearing, loss of, with, Hyosc.
>> very acute, with, Op.

Heat and shivering, with, Sabi.
>> flashes of, with, *Sep.*, *Sulph.*

Hunger and faintness at eleven A.M., Sulph.

Hysteria, from, (Cann. i.), Caul., Nux m., Sabi., Viburn. pr.

Inertia, uterine. See under Uterus.

Influenza, during epidemic, Camph.

Irritability, with, *Cham.*, *Nux v.*, Sep.
>> wishes to be alone, Nux v.

Jarring, worse from, Bell.

Labor-like pains. See under Uterine Region. Also, Repertory on Labor.

Later months, in the, Op.

Laxness of tissues, with, Sep.

Lead poisoning, from, Plb.

Legs, cramps in the, with, Rhus t., *Viburn. pr.*
>> fidgetiness of the, with, Zinc.

Legs, languor of the, Sulph.

  weakness of the, and small of back, with, K. carb.

  varices of the, with, Sep.

Leucorrhœa, from, *Calc.*, Camph., *Lyc.*, Ruta, *Sep.*, *Sulph.*

Lie down, feels that she must, K. carb.

Lifting, from. See Exertion.

Limbs. See Extremities ; also, Legs.

Lips, dry, with, Bry.

Loins, pains in the, with, Calc., Carb. v., Caul., Lyc.

  from strain in the, Cinnam.

Loquacity, unceasing, with, Stram.

Low-spirited, with, Plb.

  with weeping, *Ign.*, Lyc., *Sep.*

Mammæ, cold childs and pricking sensation in the, with, Cimic.

Menses usually too profuse and too often, Calc.

  have been pale or scanty or premature, Carb. v.

Misstep, from. See Strain.

Moaning, which seems to relieve, Bell.

Month, the. See the specified month.

  during any. Viburn. pr.

Motion, worse from, Arg. nit., Arn., Croc.

Motion, see, also, under Hæmorrhage, this
      Repertory.

    of child. See under Child.

Mouth dry, with, Bry, *Nux m.*

Move, afraid to, Acon.

    dreads to, or to be moved, Nux v.

Muscular weakness, Gels.

Narcotics, from. See Drugs.

Nausea, with, *Bry.*, Croc., Dig., *Ip.*, K. carb.,
      Phos., Verat. a.

    continuous, without a moment's relief,
      Ip.

Nervous sensibility, from, *Asar.*, Camph.,
      Fer., Plat., Sep.

Noise, sensibility to, *Bell.*, Sulph.

Nose, yellow saddle across the, Sep.

Os uteri, excrescences on; deep ulcers with
      ragged edges, Merc.

Ovarian region, stinging in the, Apis.

    pain in, especially at night, making her
      nervous and restless, Pod.

Overheating, from, Croc.

Ovum, membranes of an early, remain,
      keeping up a constant flow, China.

Pain predominating, especially, Apis, Arn.,
      Canth., Caul., Cham., Cimic., Coff.,
      Gels., K. carb., Nux v., Op., Pod.,

Puls., Rhus t., Sep., Viburn. op., Viburn. pr.

Pain. See, also, the location of the pain.

 all over, with, Bry.

 comes and goes suddenly, Bell.

 face, with fiery-red, Fer.

 hæmorrhage, without, Arn.

 hæmorrhage and, alternate, Puls.

 night, at, especially in the latter part, Rhus t.

 very severe, Viburn. pr.

Palpitation of the heart, with, Viburn. pr.

Perspiration, with cold, Dig., Verat. a.

 hot, about the head, China.

 want of, dry skin, Nux m.

Placenta, retained. See After-birth, and Repertory on Retained Placenta.

Plethora, from, Acon., Alet. far., Apis, Calc., Sabi.

Pressing down, with. See Bearing Down.

Prolapsus uteri. See Uterus, prolapsus.

Prostration, with, China.

Pulse, full and strong, with vascular activity and red face, Fer.

 imperceptible, China, Sec.

 very slow, Dig.

Quiet, desires to be, Bry

Respiration, rapid, with, Acon.

Restlessness, with, Apis, Ars., Rhus t.

    and agony, with, Cham.

    and agony, great nervousness, Pod.

Retching, with, Verat. a.

Rheumatism, from, Caul., Cimic., Rhus t.

Sadness, with, Lyc.

Second month, in, Apis, K. carb.

Sensibility of the nerves. See Nervous Sensibility.

Septicæmia after, threatened, Arn., Ars., Bapt., *Pyrog.*

Seventh month, at about the, Ruta.

Sexual organs. See Genitals.

    intercourse, from too frequent, Cann. sat.

Shocks, from. See Concussion.

Shuddering, with, Cham.

Sighing, with, *Ign.*

Sight. See Vision.

Sings, constantly, Stram.

Sit down, feels that she must, K. carb.

Skin, dry, Nux m.

    pale, loose, cold, with, Camph.

    tender and sensitive, Sep.

Sleeplessness, with, Op.

Slowly, everything seems to be done, too, Arg. nit.

Sobbing. See Weeping.

Soreness, with, *Arn.*

Spasms, with. See Convulsions.

Spasmodic pains. Nux v., Op. (See Repertory on Labor.)

Spinal affections, with, Sil.

Spitefulness, with, Cham.

Step, false. See Concussion.

Stimulants, from. See Drugs.

Stool, desire for, at every pain, Nux v

   desire for, constant, Sabi.

   desire for, often, Cham.

   frequent, but natural, Pod.

Stomach, deathly faint, sinking sensation at pit of, Dig.

   " goneness " at pit of, with, Ign.

   painful, empty, gone, feeling in pit of, with, Sep.

Strain, from, *Cinnam., Rhus t.*

Sweat. See Perspiration.

Talking, praying, etc., Stram.

Tension of body, sense of. See Constriction.

Thighs, cramp-like contractions of the, Rhus t.

Third month, at, Apis, Cimic., Croc., K. carb., Kreo., *Sabi.*, Sec., Thuj.

   month, blood black, Kreo.

Thirst, with, for large quantities of water,
    Bry.
    with, for icy-cold water, Verat. a.
Thirstlessness, with, Apis, Puls.
Throat, dry, with, Nux m.
Thunderstorm, from, Cinnam., Natr. c.,
    (Rhod.).
Time of. See the month in which it occurs.
    a short, seems very long to her, Arg. nit.
Tingling all over body, better having the
    limbs rubbed, Sec.
Toothache, with, Sep.
Turn over, afraid to, Acon.
Umbilicus, pain about the, passing off into
    the uterus, Ip.
Unconsciousness, with, China, Hyosc., Ip.
Urination painful, with, Canth, Erig., Nux v.
Urine, constant desire to pass, only a few
        drops, with burning and cutting
        pain, Canth.
    flow intermits, Con.
        profuse, with, Cham.
    profuse, colorless, with the pains, Cham.
    red sand in, with, *Lyc.*, Nux v.
    scanty, with, Apis.
    sediment adhering to the vessel, offen-
        sive, Sep.

Uterine region, colicky pain in, Bell., Calc.,
    Cham., China, Sep.

    colicky pain in, with desire to urinate,
        Cham.

    coming and going suddenly, pain in, Bell.

    cramp-like pain in, Cocc., Nux m., Vi-
        burn. pr.

    cramp-like pain in, with cutting stitches,
        Ign.

    debility in the, Caul.

    labor-like pain in, alternating with
        hæmorrhage, Cham., Puls., Sec.

    labor-like pain in, Apis, Arn., Bell.,
        Calc., Caul., Cham., Cimic., Hyosc.,
        Ip., K. carb., Lyc., Nitr. ac., Nux
        v., Op., Plat., Pod., Puls., Sabi.,
        Sec., Sep., Ustil.

    labor-like pain in, as if pelvic contents
        would issue through the vulva,
        Bell., Nitr. ac., Sep., Ustil.

    labor-like pain in, as if pelvic contents
        would issue through vulva when
        standing, Calc.

    labor-like pain in, extending into back
        and thighs, K. carb.

    labor-like pain in, extending into hypo-
        chondrion, Cham.

Uterine region, labor-like pain in, extending
    into thighs, Apis, Cham., K. carb.,
    Viburn. op.

labor-like pain in, extending into ova-
    rian region, Pod.

labor-like pain, shooting across abdo-
    men from right to left, Lyc.

labor-like pain in, spasmodic, Caul.

labor-like pain in, from urging, Arn.

motion and pain in, as of something
    alive, Croc.

pains across the, Nux v., Puls.

pain and distension in, China, Lyc.

pain in, exciting desire to defecate, or
    urinate, Nux v.

pain in, faint, sick sensation in abdo-
    men, with, Sabi.

pain in, with restlessness and heaviness,
    Cham.

pain in, shooting to legs, Viburn. op.

restlessness, great, and agony referred to
    the, Cham.

sinking, empty sensation in, Ign., Sep.

soreness in, Nux v.

tremulous sensation in, Plat.

weakness, great, in, Phos.

weight in, sense of, Alet. far.

Uterus, burning pain in, with, Bry.
    congestion of.   See Congestion.
    cramps, with cutting stitches, Ign.
    difficult contractions of, after, Sec.
    displacement of, subject to, Trill.
    enlarged, Ustil.
    hard lump on neck of, Kreo.
    inertia of, from, Alet. far., Caul., China,
        Cimic., Fer., Helon., Puls., Sabi.,
        Sec., Ustil.
    non-development of, abortion from, Plb.
    prolapsus, with, Alet. far., Erig., Pod.
    prolapsus of, and of rectum, Pod.
    prolapsus of, after, Kreo., Pod.
    retained after-birth. See After-birth.
    subinvolution of, Cimic.
    ulceration of, from, Canth, Helon.
    weight in, sense of, Alet. far.
Vagina, dryness in, sense of, Lyc.
    pressing-down feeling in, Sil.
Vertigo, with, Calc., Cham., Con.
    great, when turning the head in bed, Con.
    on rising from a recumbent position ;
        she has to lie down again, Acon.
    when going up-stairs, Calc.
    when stooping or rising from stooping,
        Bell.

Vision, loss of, with, Hyosc.

Vomiting, with, Cocc., Dig., K. carb., Phos.,
Sulph., Verat. a.

bilious, Cocc.

of ingesta, Sabi., Sulph.

Vulva, and mons veneris, feel cold and sensitive to touch, Plat.

itching of the, Lyc.

itching of the, with soreness, Sep., Sulph.

trembling sensation from, into abdomen, Plat.

swelling of, and inguinal glands, Merc.

varices, Carb. v.

Weakness, with, Alet. far., Fer., Helon.,
Sulph.

Weeping, with, *Ign.*, Lyc., Sep.

Women, delicate, anæmic, Trill.

dysmenorrhœa, who have a history of,
Viburn. pr.

feeble, who have borne many children,
in, Sec.

leucophlegmatic, in, Calc.

tall, slender, in, Phos.

scrawny, sallow, in, Sec.

weak, in, Goss., Helon., Sec.

Wrench, from a, Rhus t.

Yawning, with, Apis, Cham.

HÆMORRHAGE.

ABDOMEN, alive, sensation of something in, Croc.

convulsive jerks across the, China.

cutting across the, from right to left, better by flow of blood, Lyc.

cutting pain in, Iod.

cutting pain about the umbilicus, with, Ip.

cutting pain deep in lower, extending to back, Croc.

distension of, with, China., Nux m.

distension of, with intermitting flow, China.

dragging pain from, to back, with, Carbo v.

drawing pain in the, Sep.

heaviness in, with, Apis.

painful sense of weakness, and sense of coldness and emptiness across the, Phos.

rumbling in, with, Lyc., Nux m.

sensitive, very, and painful to touch, Phos.

stitches, sharp, darting from the, to vagina, Kreo.

string pulling, to back, sense of, Plb.

Abdomen, tension in, painful, China.

Abortion. See Repertory on Abortion, under
       Discharge and Hæmorrhage.

    after (especially), Bell., Cham., *China*,
        Cinnam., *Croc.*, Erig., *Fer.*, Hyosc.,
        Ip., K. carb., Lyc., Nitr. ac., Plat.,
        Sabi., *Sec.*, Sil., Trill.

    profuse during (especially), Arn., Cham.,
        Ip., Puls., Sabi., Sep., Sec., Viburn.
        op., Viburn. pr.

Active, Acet. ac., Acon., Apis, Arn., Bell.,
        Calc., Cham., China, Cinnam., Coff.,
        Croc., Fer., Ham., Hyosc., Ign., Ip.,
        Phos., Plat., Sec., Trill., Ustil.

After-birth. See Placenta.

After-pains, profuse between the, *Bell.*

Air, desire for fresh, by having doors and
        windows open, Puls., Sec.

Alternating with labor-pains, Puls.

Anæmia, from, Cinnam., Ham., K. carb.

Anger, after, *Cham.*, (Staph.).

Anus, itching of, with, Carb. v.
    prolapsus of, with, Pod.
    sense of weight in, like a ball, Sep.

Anxiety, with, Acon., Ham.

Appearance, of various, Carb. v.

Appearing suddenly, dark, Ars.
        suddenly and ceasing as suddenly, Bell.

Apthæ, with, Ars.

Atony.   See under Uterine.

Back, dragging in, worse laughing or moving, Phos.

> heat running up the, a feeling of intense, Phos.

> pain all the way from sacrum to pubes, Sabi.

> pain from, to uterus, Helon.

> pain in, Bry., Cimic.

> pain in, as if it would break, Bell.

> pain in, extending down over the buttocks, K. carb.

> pain in, extending into both groins, Plat.

> pain in, with profuse flow, Trill.

> pain in small of, Iod.

> pain in small of, as if broken, Phos.

> pain in small of, through hips and down thighs, Nitr. ac.

Bearing-down pain, profuse with easy flow, Cycl.

> down, with, *Bell.*, Cham., Cimic., Kreo., *Lac. c.*, *Sec.*

> down, violent, as if pelvic contents would issue through vulva., Nitr. ac.

Bed, feels too hot, Op.

> feels very hard, Bell., Pyrog.

Bed, worse when getting out, Ip.

Belching, with relief, Arg. nit., K. carb.

Black blood, Cham., China, Croc., Fer., Kreo.,
Plat., Puls., Sec., Sulph.

clotted, Cham., China, Croc., *Fer.*, *Lyc.*,
Puls., Sabi.

liquid, *Sec.*

offensive, Cham., Croc., Kreo., Sec.

partly coagulated, thin, profuse, Fer.

stringy, *Croc.*

thick, not coagulated, Plat.

thick, tarry mass, Plat.

Bladder, irritation of neck of, great, Canth.,
Erig.

Body, feels as if growing larger in every
direction, Plat.

Bones, feel as if broken, Trill.

Breath, gasping for, as if panting, Ip., Laur.

Breathing, difficult, with, Acet. ac., Carb. v.,
China., Ip.

labored, Fer., Ip.

rapidly, Fer.

Bright-red flow, Arn., *Bell.*, *Calc.*, *Cinnam.*,
Erig., Fer., Ham., *Hyosc.*, *Ip.*, Lac.
c., Lyc., *Millef.*, Nitr. ac., Nux v.,
Pyrog., Rhus t., *Sabi.*, Sec., *Trill.*,
Ustil., Viburn. pr.

Bright-red flow, clots, with, Trill.

> continuous, *Hyosc.*, *Ip.*, *Millef.*
>
> hot, *Bell.*, Lac. c.
>
> lumpy, Arn., Ustil.
>
> lumpy in paroxysms with colic, Bell., Nux v., Rhus t.
>
> partly clotted, *Sabi.*
>
> partly fluid and partly clotted, Ustil.
>
> profuse, at the least motion, Trill.

Brown fluid, Apocyn. c., Sec.

Cause, from the least (Ambr.), Sep.

Ceases suddenly and suddenly returns, Bell.

> for a few moments, then renews with redoubled force, Puls.

Cervix uteri, darting pains in, from below upward, Sep.

Chamomile, after a dose of, *China*, Ign.

Changeable in character, Puls.

Chest, burning pain in, with, Carbo v.

> great weakness in, speech difficult, Stann.

Chilliness, with, Fer., Ip.

Clots. See, also, Coagulated.

> with, Cham., China, Cimic., Ip., Nux v., Puls., Pyrog., Rhus t., Sabi., Stram., Ustil.
>
> dark, *Cham.*, *China*, Puls., Sabi., Ustil.

Clots, dark, alternating with bloody serum, Plb.

    dark, in paroxysms, Puls.

    hard and black, mixed with fluid blood passing away in a dark, tarry mass, Plat.

    large, Apocyn. c., Arn., Coff, Stram.

    large black, Arn., *Coff.*, Sec.

    large in bright-red blood, Arn., Bell., Sabi., Ustil.

    large, mixed with pale, watery blood, China.

    large, offensive, Bell., Kreo.

    large, with volent pain; increased by motion, Arg. nit.

    partly bright-red and partly bloody serum, Lyc.

Coagula, from retained, Puls.

Coagulated. See Clots, and the color of flow.

    Apocyn. c., Arn., Bell., Cham., China, Coff., Croc., Fer., Kreo., Lyc., Nux v., Plat., Puls., Rhus t., Sabi., Sec., Stram., Trill.

    with profuse dark flow, Trill.

    with profuse, thin, partly black, flow, Fer.

Coagulating easily, Fer., Lac. c.

    speedily, profuse, hot, with retained placenta, *Bell.*

Coffea, after abuse of, Nux v.

Coition, after, Arn.

Cold paroxysms, icy, and flushes of heat, Sep.

Coldness, with, Acet. ac., Carb. v., China, Ip., Laur., Sec., Sep.

Colic, with, Fer., Nux m., Nux v., Rhus t.

Coma, with, China, Crotal., Laur.

Concussions, falls, shocks, after, Arn., Cinnam., Puls., Rhus t., Ruta., Sulph.

Confinement, after. See Labor, after.

Confusion, with. See Head.

Constipation, from high living, etc., Nux v.

    consult Repertory on Abortion.

Continuous flow, Apocyn. c., Arn., Carb. v., Ham., *Hyosc.*, *Ip.*, Millef., Phos., Sec., Ustil.

    but slow, *Ham.*, Ustil.

    or in paroxysms, Apocyn. c.

    profuse, IP.

    see, also, under the color of the flow.

Convulsions. See Spasms, and Repertory on Convulsions.

Convulsive discharge, Cham.

Covered, will not be, Sec.

Dancing, after, with or without pain, Croc.

Dark flow, Apis, Ars., Bell., Bry., Canth., Cham., China, Cimic., Cocc., Croc., Crotal., Ham., Helon., Kreo., Nitr. ac., Nux m., Plb., Puls., Sabi., Sec., Sulph. ac., Trill.

    blackish clots in thin watery blood, Sabi.

    coagulated, occasionally interrupted by bright-red gushes, Cham.

    clotted, profuse for days, Trill.

    clots. See under Clots.

    fluid, Bry., Crotal., Plat., *Sec.*

    oozing, with small coagula for days, Ustil.

    or bright, clotted or fluid, profuse in equal parts of, *Sabi.*

    painless, immediately after labor, Nux m., Plat.

    profuse, Sep.

    profuse, clotted, Trill.

    profuse at first, then for a few days bloody ichor with pungent odor, corrosive itching and smarting of parts, Kreo.

    red, with pain in back and splitting headache, Bry.

Dark red, with very dark clots in thin, watery
           blood, Sabi.
    semi-fluid, but not watery, Ustil.
    suddenly appearing, Ars.
    thick, *Nux m.*, Plat.

Death, fear of, with Acon., Coff., Nux m.

Debility, from general, Alet. far., Ars., Caul.,
           China, Fer.
    with. See Exhaustion.

Delirium, with, Hyosc., Sec., Stram.

Delivery, after. See Labor, after.

Depression, with mental, Ign., Nux v., Plb.

Despair, with, Coff.

Despondency, with, Ign.

Dizziness. See Vertigo.

Dropsy, complicated with, Apocyn. c.

Drugs, abuse of, after, Nux v.

Dyspnœa. See Breathing, difficult.

Ears, ringing in the, China.

Emotions, from violent, Acon., Bell., Bry.,
           Cham., Cocc., Croc., Hyosc., Phos.,
           Plat., Puls., Sep., Stram., Sulph.

Excitement, mental, from, Calc., Ign., Nux v.
    mental, with, Acon., Croc., Hyosc.
    vascular, with, Hyosc., Pyrog.

Exertion, after great, Cinnam., Helon., Mil-
           lef., Nitr. ac., Nux v.
    after mental, Plat.

Exhaustion, with, Ars., Carb. v., Caul.,
    China, Coff., Erig., Ham., Ip., Sabi.,
    Sec., Sulph.

    from loss of much blood, *China*, Chin.
    s., Erig., Laur., Trill.

Expansion of body in every direction, sen-
    sation of, with, Plat.

Extremities, cold, China, Laur., Trill.

    feels better when drawing up the, Sep.

    pains in the, Cimic., Stram.

    weakness of, with, Sabi.

Eyes, congested, with, Bell.

    dimness of vision, with, Laur.

    sees persons or objects on closing the,
    China.

Face, fiery red, with, Fer.

    hot, red, with, Bell.

    pale and bluish, with, China.

    pale. See Paleness.

    sallow, with, Helon.

    yellow spots on, with, Sep.

Faintness, with, Apis, Apocyn. c., Bry.,
    China, Croc., Ip., Kreo., Lyc., Nux
    m., Sulph.

Falls, after. See Concussions.

False step. See Strain.

Fanned, desire to be, Carb. v., China.

Fatigue, with, Arn.

Fear of death. See Death, fear of.

  moving or turning, of, Acon.

  that something will surely happen, Acon.

Feet, cold, damp, with, Calc.

  cold, with, Croc., Sep., Sulph.

Fifth month to the seventh, Sep.

Fingers, hold them apart, and is greatly concerned about it, Sec.

First month, in, from overheating, Croc.

Flatulency, with, Lyc., Nux m.

Fluid blood. See Thin, and under color of blood.

Fluids, from loss of, *China.*

Fœtid blood, Cham., Croc., Sec., Trill.

  see, also, offensive.

Formication or tingling over body, with desire to have limbs rubbed, followed by unconsciousness and cold condition, Sec.

Frequent attacks, almost well, then returns, Krec., Nux v., Sulph.

Fright, after, Acon., Bell., Nux v., Op., Sec.

  after, when the fear remains, Acon.

Frightened, seems to be, Stram.

Genitals, sensitiveness of the, Coff., *Plat.*

Genitals, urging toward, painful, Kreo.

Giddiness. See Vertigo.

Grief, full of suppressed, Ign.

Groin, pain in, Coff., Sep.

Gushes in, Cham., China, Ip., Lac. can., Puls., Sabi., Sec., Trill., Ustil., Viburn. op.

    in, at every effort to vomit, profuse; gasping for breath, IP.

        in, comes suddenly, and then stops again, Erig.

    in, profuse, Ham., IP., Viburn op.

Hands, pale and bluish, China.

Hatred, from Apis.

Headache, with, Fer., Glon., Ip.

    hammering, especially about the temples, Ham.

    splitting, Bry.

Head, confusion of, Apocyn. c., Crotal.

    Congested, Bell., Ip.

    dulness of, Apocyn. c.

    heat on vertex, Sulph

    heaviness of, China.

    hot, body cool, Arn.

    lifts the, from pillow frequently, starts up as if in a fright, Stram.

    nervousness and weakness in, Sabi.

Head, tearing in the vertex, Laur.
    throbbing in, Bell., Croc.
Heart, anxiety about the, Plb.
    palpitation of, Apocyn. c., Croc.
    suffocative spells around the, peculiar,
        Laur.
Heat, flushes of, Sep., Sulph.
Heating, over, from, Croc., Nitr. ac.
Hot blood, *Bell.*, *Lac. can.*
Hungry spells, gets, Sulph.
Hysteria, subjects of, Hyosc., Nux m.
Inertia of uterus.   See under Uterine.
Intermitting flow, Apocyn. c., Cham., China,
        Erig., Kreo., Nux v., Phos., Sabi.,
        Sec., Sulph., Ustil.
    alternating with labor-pains, Puls.
    ceases for a few moments, then renews
        with redoubled force, Puls.
    pouring out freely, then ceasing for a
        short time, Phos.
    with uterine cramps, colic and pain-
        ful distension of abdomen, China.
Irritability, with, Hyosc., Nux v.
Jar, worse from the least, Bell.
Jealousy, from, Apis.
Jerking.   See Twitching.
    flow worse from, Hyosc.

Joints, pain in, with, Sabi.

Labor, after (especially), Acet. ac., *Arn.*,
            Bell., Bry., Caul., Cham., *China,*
            Cinnam., *Croc.*, Erig., *Fer.*, Ham.,
            Hyosc., *Ip.*, K. carb., Kreo., Lach.,
            Millef., Nitr. ac., Nux m., Nux v.,
            Plat., *Sabi.*, *Sec.*, (Senec.), *Trill.*,
            Ustil.

   days and weeks, after, K. carb.

   difficult, after, Phos.

   hasty, after, *Caul.*

   instrumental, after, Arn.

   protracted, after, Arn., Sec.

   protracted, from uterine atony, after, *Sec.*

Labor, during (especially), *Bell.*, Cham.,
            China, *Cinnam.*, Fer., Hyosc., *Ip.*,
            Lyc., Plat., *Sabi.*, *Sec.*

Labor-pains, alternating with flow, Puls.

   after first few in primiparæ, Cinnam.

   cease from hæmorrhage, Cimic.

   violent, Cham.

   like. See Pains.

Legs, pains in, Cimic.

   tearing pains in, with, Cham.

Leucorrhœa, after, Mag. mur., Sabi., Iod.

Lifting from. (See Strain), Cinnam., Croc.,
            Helon., *Pod.*, Rhus t.

Light, worse from, Bell.

Limbs. See Extremities.

Lips, dry, with, Bry.
    pale, with, Fer.

Liquid blood. See under Thin, and the
        color of blood.

Loins, pains in the, Fer., Iod.
    strain in, from, Cinnam., Croc.

Loquacity, with, Sec., *Stram.*

Lumpy. See Clots, and the color of the
        blood.

Lying down, worse, Kreo.

Mammæ, acute pain in the, Iod.

Mania, with Hyosc.

Menses, too frequent and too profuse, Calc.

Mental excitement. See Excitement.
    depression, Ign., Nux v.

Motion, worse from, Arg. nit., Bell., *Bry.*,
        Calc., Coff., *Croc.*, *Erig.*, Plb., *Sabi.*,
        Sec., *Trill.*, Ustil.
    brought on from slightest, *Croc.*, *Sabi.*
    profuse bright-red from least, Trill.
    worse from least, but better from walk-
        ing about, *Sabi.*
    worse from slightest, of any part of
        body, even hands, Bry.

Mouth, dry, with, Bry., Nux m.

Nausea, with, Apocyn. c., Arn., Bry., IP.

Noise, worse from, Bell.

Nose, yellow saddle across, Sep.

Nursing, while, the child, Sil.

Offensive. See Fœtid, also.

    Bell., Cham., Croc., Crotal., Kreo., Sabi., Sec., Ustil.

    pungent, Kreo.

    putrid, Cham.

Oozing, dark, with small coagula for days, Ustil.

Os uteri, ulcers on, Nitr. ac.

Ovarian region, paroxysms of pain in right, extending toward uterus, Lach.

    region, stinging sensation in, Apis.

Ovaries congested, Iod.

    pain in, alternating from side to side, Lac. can.

Pain, lancinating, burning, Ars.

    labor-like, with, Cimic., Fer., Lyc., Rhus t.

    stitching, with, K. carb.

    with or without, Arn., Cinnam.

Painless (Bov.), Calc., Croc., Ham., (Magn. c.), Millef., Nux m., Plat., Sabi., Sec.

Pale blood, Carb. v., China, Fer., Hyosc., Merc., Millef., Sabi.

    consult, also, Watery.

Pale blood, clotted, very thin, offensive;
  worse from motion, Sabi.
  mixed with large black clots, Arn.
  with pale lips and face, Fer.
Paleness, with, Acet. ac., Carb. v., Fer., Ip.,
  Laur., Plb.
Palpitation. See under Heart.
Paroxysms, in, Apocyn. c., Bell., China,
  Nux v., Puls., Rhus t., Sabi.
Passive flow, Acet. ac., Alet. far., Carb. v.,
  Caul., China, Chin. s., Cimic., Cin-
  nam., *Croc.*, *Ham.*, Plb., *Sec.*, *Sulph.
  ac.*, Ustil., Visc. alb.
Periodical, Arg. nit., Ip.
Perspiration, cold, with, Ip., Laur.
Placenta, after removal of the, Bell., Cin-
  nam., IP., Puls., Sec.
  retained, or coagula, from, Puls.
  retained, from, Bell., Canth., Caul.,
   Puls., Sabi., Sec., Sep., Stram.
  retained, from, with delirium, Sec.,
   Stram.
  retained, from, profuse speedily coagu-
   lating blood, *Bell.*
Plethora, with, Acon.
Pregnancy, during, Cocc., Croc., K. carb.,
  Kreo., Phos., Plat., Rhus t., Sabi., Sep.

Pregnancy, fifth to seventh month of, Sep.
      second month of, Apis, K. carb.
      third month of, Croc., *K. carb.*, Kreo.,
        Sabi.
Pressure downward. See Bearing Down.
Primiparæ, severe in, after first few pains,
      Cinnam.
Profuse flow, Acon., Apis, Apocyn. c., Arg.
      nit., Arn., *Bell.*, *Bry.*, Calc., *Caul.*,
      Cham., China, Cimic., *Cinnam.*,
      Croc., Erig., Fer., Glon., *Ham.*,
      Helon., Hyosc., K. carb., Kreo.,
      IP., Lyc., Millef., Nitr. ac., *Nux v.*,
      Phos., Puls., *Sabi.*, *Sec.*, Trill., Vi-
      burn. op.
    between the after-pains, Bell.
    continuous, Hyosc., *IP.*
    equal parts clotted or fluid, dark or
        bright, Sabi.
    in gushes, Ham., Ip., Viburn. op.
    long-lasting, Phos.
    sudden, Bell., *Cinnam.*
    thin, partly black, coagulated, Fer.
    see, also, under the color of blood.
Prostration. See Exhaustion.
Pulse, feeble, with, Apocyn. c., Carb. v.,
      China, Ip., Kreo.

Pulse, full, bounding, Bell.

    full, hard, Fer.

      quick, with Apocyn. c., Carb. v., Pyrog. Sec.

Pungent, Kreo.

Putrid, Cham.

Quiet, may be kept in check to a certain extent by remaining perfectly, Erig.

Quinine, after, Fer., *Ip.*, Nux v., Puls.

Rectum, irritation of the, with, Erig.

    pressure over the, with, Ip.

Restlessness, with, Apis, Op., Pyrog.

    death-like, Pyrog.

Rising up in bed, worse from, Acon.

      up in bed, fainting from, Apocyn. c., Bry.

      up, flow better, Kreo.

Sacrum, burning pain across, with, Carb. v.

      forcing-down pain from, to pubes, Sabi.

      separated, sensation as if, Cham.

Scanty flow, Cocc., Nux v., Thuj.

    compare Pain predominating, in Repertory on Abortion.

Second month, at the, Apis, K. carb.

Sensation as if the body were growing larger in every direction, with the flowing, Plat.

Sexual organs. See Genitals and Vulva.
 excitement, great, Plat., Stram.
Shuddering, with, Fer., Ip.
Sighing, with, Ign.
Singing, praying, etc., Stram.
Sit up, cannot, in bed, Acon.
Skin, blueness of, China.
 dry, pale, yellowish, Plb.
 red spots, like bee stings, on, Apis.
Sleep. See Coma.
Sleeplessness, with, Nux m.
Sleepy, but cannot sleep, Bell., Op.
Slow, everything done seems too, Arg. nit.
Sobbing, with, Ign.
Sopor. See Coma.
Spasms, hysterical, with, Cimic.
 with, Hyosc.
Speaking, worse from, Bry.
Step, false. See Strain.
Stinging sensation over body, Apis.
Stool, after every, Ind., Lyc.
 frequent calls to, with, Nux v.
Stomach, faint feeling at pit of, Ign.
 irritability of, great, Apocyn. c.
 painful, empty, gone feeling in pit of,
  Sep.
 saucer-bottom swelling in pit of, Calc.

Stomach, sinking in the, Trill.

Strain, from, *Cinnam.*, Croc., Rhus t.
    see Lifting.

Stringy, Apocyn. c., *Croc.*, Lac can., Ustil.
    see, also, under the color of blood.

Suddenly appearing, dark, Ars.
    appearing, Cinnam., Erig., Millef.
    ceasing and as suddenly returning,
      Bell.

Sweat. See Perspiration.

Talking. See Speaking.

Tendency, hæmorrhagic, of a, Fer.

Thick flow, Carb. v., *Nux m.*, Plat., Puls.,
    Sulph., Trill.
    see, also, the color of blood.

Thin, fluid flow, Apocyn. c., Bry., China,
    Crotal., Fer., Kreo., Lyc., Millef.,
    Nitr. ac., Plat., Plb., Puls., Sabi.,
    Sec., Sulph. ac.
    mixed with coagula, China., Fer., Kreo.,
      Sabi., Sec.
    see under the color of blood, also.

Third month, at, Croc., *K. carb.*, Kreo., *Sabi.*,
    Thuj.

Thirst, with, Acet. ac., Bry., Fer.

Thoughts, her, horrify her, Plat.

Throat, sensation as if full up to the, Lyc.

Time, a short, seems very long to her, Arg.
 nit.

Tingling. See Formication.

Trembling weakness felt over entire body,
 Caul.

 sensation of, all over, without actual
  trembling, Sulph. ac.

Twitching of the muscles, China.

 of the limbs, Hyosc.

Umbilicus, cutting pain about the, Ip.

Unconsciousness, with, China, Sec.

Urinary complications, with, Apocyn. c.

Urination, constant desire to, almost, Canth.

 frequent urging to, China.

 painful, with, Canth., Erig.

Urine, colorless, frequent discharge of, Cham.

 hot, Fer.

 offensive, with sediment adhering to
  vessel, Sep.

Uterine cramps, with, China.

 inertia, with, Caul., China, Puls., Sabi.,
  Sec., Ustil.

 region, bruised and sore feeling in the,
  Arn.

 region, weight in the, Alet. far., Sep.

Uterus, colic of, China.

 congested, with, Iod., Sep.

Uterus, contracted into little lumps, felt through abdominal walls, Cham.

cramps of, with, China.

darting pain in cervix, upward, Sep.

distinct pressure in, as if something would come out, Ant. cr.

expulsion of flatus from, Nux m.

feebly contracted, Caul., Nux m.

hard, somewhat, Laur.

labor-pains, violent, in, Cham.

pressure over the, violent, with, Ip., Sep.

prolapse of, Pod.

scirrhus of neck and vagina, Kreo.

soft and relaxed, Caul., Laur.

spasms of, China.

subinvoluted, blood imprisoned in the, causing gradual dilatation, Kreo.

weight in, sense of, Sep.

Vagina, flatus from, Nux m.

scirrhus of, Kreo.

Vanishing of the senses, China.

Varicose veins, knotty, swollen, painful, Ham.

Vertigo, with, Acon., Calc., China, Crotal., Fer., Ip.

Viscid, Croc.

Vision. See Eyes.

Visions of rats, mice, vermin, etc., Stram.

Vomiting, with, Apocyn. c., Ip.

    profuse flow with every effort at, IP.

Vulva, itching of, Carb. v., Coff., Kreo.

Walking after, with or without pain, Croc.

    better from, Sabi.

Warmth, better from, K. carb.

Watery, flow, China, Fer., Puls.

    see, also, Pale.

    large clots mixed with pale, China.

    pale, with coagula, China, Sabi.

Weakness. See Debility and Exhaustion.

Weeping, with, Ign., Phos.

Women, broken-down constitution, of a, Crotal.

    cachectic, Nitr. ac., Sec.

    delicate, thin, Iod., K. carb.

    given to reveries, Puls.

    habitually flood after every parturition, who, *Trill.*

    high living, who have, Nux v.

    lungs, hæmorrhage from, subject to, Millef.

    mild, tearful, Puls.

    obesity, inclined to, with lax muscles and skin, Hyosc.

    phlegmatic, Calc.

Women, phthisical, Millef., Phos.
 plethoric, Acon., Bell., Calc.
 rheumatic, Ant. cr., Bry., Caul., Cimic.,
  Rhus t.
 sedentary habits, of, Nux v.
 scrawny, Sec.
 subject to profuse menses, Calc.
 tall, slender, Phos.
 weakly, Fer.
Yawning, with, Apis.

RETAINED PLACENTA.

This Repertory is necessarily brief. Any remedy may be indicated. Prescribe on the prominent symptoms, or the character of the flow when present. Consult Repertory on Labor for pains and other symptoms, and that on Hæmorrhage for the character of the flow. When *no* symptoms are present, *Sepia* after abortion and *Pulsatilla* after labor, are highly recommended by good authority.

ABDOMEN, burning pain in lower, Canth.
 cutting pain in lower, usually running
  upward, or upward and backward,
  Gels.

Abdomen, labor-like pains in, Fer.

    motion in, slight sensation of, Sabi.

    redness and soreness of lower external,
        with retention of urine, Puls.

    sensitiveness of the, Canth.

Abortion, after (especially), Goss., Sec., Sep.

Adherent. See Placenta.

Air, desire for fresh, Puls., Sec.

Anguish, with, Canth.

Back, burning pain in, Canth.

    pain from, to pubes, *Sabi.*

Bearing down, constant, sense of, *Sec.*

Breath, desire to draw a long, Croc.

Contractions of uterus absent, Caul., Cimic.,
        Puls.

    pains deficient, Ip., *Puls.*, Sec.

    pains imperfect or else very prolonged,
        Sec.

    pains out of proportion to the, Coff.

Convulsions, with, Canth.

    see, also, Repertory on Convulsions.

Covered, averse to being, Sec.

Death, fear of, Acon., Coff.

Delirium, with, Stram.

Distress, with, Bell., Canth., Cimic., *Coff.*, Ip.,
        Sec.

Dryness of the surface of the body, Bell.

Eyes, injected, with, Bell.

Eyeballs, pain in the, Cimic.

Exhaustion, from, Caul.

    with, Sulph.

Extremities, cold, Croc., Sep.

    paroxysms of pain extending down posterior surface of, Rhus t.

Face, red, with, Bell., Fer.

Faintness, with, Croc., Sulph.

Fanned, wants to be, Sulph.

Feet, cramps in the, Cupr.

Feverishness, with, Bell., Canth.

Flooding, with. See Hæmorrhage.

Genitals, external, very sensitive, Plat.

Hæmorrhage. See Repertory on Hæmorrhage.

    bright red, with, IP.

    in large clots, or stringy, Croc.

    intermitting with, Puls.

    oozing of dark grumous blood, Plat.

    partly fluid and partly clotted, Fer., *Sabi.*

    passive, with, Sec.

    profuse, of hot blood, speedily coagulating, Bell.

    with (especially), Bell., Caul., China, *Croc.*, Fer., *Ip.*, Plat., *Puls.*, Sabi., Sec., Stram., Visc. alb.

Hands, cramps in, with, Cupr.

Head, brain feels too large for skull, Cimic.

Headache, with, Cimic., Fer.

Heart, palpitation of, Croc.

Heat, flushes of, Sep., Sulph.

  of surface of body, Bell.

Hour-glass contractions. See same in Repertory on Labor.

Jar, slight, causes suffering, Bell.

Labor-pains. See Contractions.

Loins, labor-like pains in the, Fer.

Moaning, with, Bell.

Nausea, with, Ip.

Pains. See Repertory on Labor.

  distressing. See Distress.

  extending down posterior surface of
   thighs, paroxysms of, Rhus t.

  extreme constrictive, impede expulsion,
   Nux v.

  imperfect, very, or else prolonged contractions, Sec.

  out of proportion to the uterine contractions, Coff.

  very intense, Sabi.

 Palpitation. See Heart.

Placenta adheres firmly, force will hardly
  dislodge it, Goss.

Placenta, adherent, Goss., Puls.

 retained or incarcerated, Visc. alb.

 retained, *Bell.*, *Canth.*, *Caul.*, Cimic.,
  Gels., Goss., PULS., *Sabi.*, *Sec.*, SEP.,
  Visc. alb.

 retained, spasmodically, Caul.

Pulse, full, hard, Fer.

 weak or none, Croc.

Restlessness, with, Puls., Rhus t.

Retained. See Placenta.

Sacrum to pubes, pains in, *Sabi.*

Shuddering, with, Fer.

Sleeplessness, with, Coff.

Sleepy, but cannot sleep, Bell., Coff.

Soreness, with, Cimic.

Spasmodic retention, Caul.

Thirstlessness, with, Puls.

Umbilicus, sharp, pinching pains about,
  running to uterus, Ip.

Urination, burning on, with, Canth.

 retention of, with redness and soreness
  of external hypogastrium, Puls.

 smarting in urethra after, Lil. t.

 teasing to, with, *Canth.*

Uterine region, cramping pains in, Plat.

 distressing, tearing pains in, Cimic.

Uterus. See, also, Contractions.

Uterus, cramps in the, Cupr.

    dilated and soft, Croc.

    neuralgia in and around, Lil. t.

    relaxed, no action, Sec.

    sharp, shooting pains in cervix, at times
        with burning, Sep.

    swelling of lips of the os, Canth.

    want of expulsive power, *Puls.*

Vagina, heat and dryness of, with, Bell.

Vertigo, with, Fer.

Vomiting, with, Canth., Ip.

Vulva. See Genitals.

Warmth, distressed by, Sec.

Weakness. See Exhaustion.

Weeping because the labor is not com-
        pleted, *Puls.*

Women, constitution of. See under Reper-
        tory on Hæmorrhage.

CONVULSIONS.

The Repertory on Labor should be consulted under most of the rubrics, as many
irregularities of labor cause convulsions. A
timely prescription will prevent this dire
calamity. Here special indications are
given. When hæmorrhage is present con-

sult Repertory on Hæmorrhage. Also with Retained Placenta and After-pains.

ABDOMEN, bloating of the, with, Merc., Mosch.

    cramps in, with, Cupr.

    distressing pains in, from before backward and upward, Gels.

    rumbling in, with, Cic., Mosch.

    sharp pains across, with, Cimic.

    tenderness of, with, Bry., Cupr.

    tympanitis, of, after labor, with, Arn.

Air, must have fresh, Carb. v., Puls.

Anæmia, from, Chlorof., Zinc.

Anger, from, Cham., Nux v., Op.

Anguish, with, Acon., Hyosc., K. brom., Lyc.

Anxiety, extreme, before, Œnan.

Apprehension, with, Crotal.

Arms, flexing and jerking the, rigidity alternates with, Ip.

    throwing about of the, Lyc.

Arouses suddenly, followed by convulsions and rigidity, Ars.

Back, burning pain in, with, Cupr.

    convulsions in, with throwing back of head, stiffness of body, tetanic, Cham.

Back, heat rushes up, to head, previous to,
    Phos.
    languor in, great, with, Nux m.
    muscles of, affected, with, Hyd. ac.
    thrown up, by limbs being forcibly
        curved, with, Hyosc.
Belching, with, Cic.
    marked relief from, which comes up in
        a torrent, Arg. nit.
    with relief from, or spasms passing off
        by frequent, K. carb.
Bent backward.   See Opisthotonos.
Between convulsions. See Interval between.
Biting, etc., with, Bell., Cupr.
Brain, compressed sensation of, a strange,
        with, Ign.
    stupefying pressure on the, with, Mosch.
    consult under Head.
Breath, cold, with, Carb. v.
Breathing, anxious, with, Ars.
    arrest of, sudden, with, Plat.
    difficult, with, Ars., Caust., Chin. s.,
        Cupr., Hyd. ac., Hyosc., Laur.,
        Œnan., Plat., Puls.
    hurried, with, Œnan.
    interruptions, frequent, with, *Cic.*
    irregular, with, Hyd. ac.

Breathing, short, with, Ars., Carb. v.

    spasms alternate with dyspnœa and suffocation, Plat.

    stertorous, continuing from one spasm to another, Op.

    suffocative, with, Hyosc., Laur., Op.

Bright light, renewal from, Canth., Nux v., *Stram.*

Carotids, pulsations of, with, *Bell.*, China, *Glon.*

    distended, with, Chin. s.

Cervix uteri, cutting pains in, thence upward, with, Gels.

Cheeks, one red the other pale, with, Cham.

Chest, oppression of, with, Hyosc.

Child, pressure of, from, on pelvic nerves or against undilating os, K. brom.

Chilliness, with, Ars.

Coldness after, with, K. phos., Laur.

Collapse, with, Carb. v., Verat. a.

Coma, with, Atrop., Bell., Crotal., *Hyosc.*, Laur., Nux v., Œnan., *Op.*, Zinc.

    consult Consciousness, loss of.

Consciousness, with, K. carb., Nux v.

    loss of, with, Arn., Ars., Atrop., Bell., Chin. s., Cic., Gels., Glon., Hyosc., Lyc., Œnan., Puls., Stram., Verat. vir.

Consciousness, loss of, continuous, lies in a
    deep sleep, Verat. vir.
    semi, with, Bell.
Contortions of upper part of body and
    limbs, during, Cic.
Convulsions have ceased, after, with full,
    hard pulse, abdominal tenderness,
    etc., Bry.
Cramps, with, Cimic., *Cupr.*
    spasms begin as. in fingers, toes and ex-
    tremities, Cupr.
Crying out. See Shrieks.
Dazed appearance, with, Bell.
Death, fear of, with, Acon.
Deglutition, difficult, with, Bell., Cupr.
Delirium, with, Crotal., *Hyosc.*, Œnan.,
    Verat. a., *Verat. vir.*, Zinc.
Delivery, after. See Labor, after.
Delusions, with, Stram.
    thinks herself possessed of beautiful
    things, Sulph.
Diarrhœa, with, Ars.
Drowsiness. See Sleepiness.
Electric shocks. See Shocks.
Emotions, after sudden, especially pleasing
    ones, Coff.
    violent, from, Ign., Nux v., Op., Verat.
    a., Verat. vir.

Epigastrium, begins with an aura in the, Nux v.

Eruptions, recently disappeared, where, Zinc.

Escape, tries to, Stram.

Excitability, mental, preceded by, Cimic.

    nervous, from, *Cimic.*, Cocc., *Coff.*, Hyosc., K. brom., K. Phos., Plat.

    spiteful, with, Cham.

    vascular, with, (Pyrog.), Verat. vir.

Exhaustion, weakness, with, *Ars.*, Carb. v., Caul., Cic., Cimic., Crotal., Gels., *Hyd. ac.*, K. Phos., Lach., Laur., Mag. phos., Verat. a.

Expansion, general, sensation of, with, *Arg. nit.*, K. brom., *Plat.*

Extremities, alternate extension and contraction of, with, Lyc.

    clammy, with, Ars.

    clonic spasms of all the, with, Laur.

    cold, with, Ars., Carb. v., Caust., Coff., Lach.

    convulsive movements of, with, Bell., Caust., China, Chin. s., Merc. c., Merc.

    forcibly curved, and the body thrown up from bed, with, Hyosc.

    lower, particularly violent, in the, Lach.

    mostly in the, Merc.

Extremities, numbness of, with, Acon.

    restlessness of, with, Atrop., Zinc.

    spreading out of the, with, Cupr.

    stretching of, commencing with, and groaning, Ign.

    stiffness of, with, Mag. phos.

    tingling in, with, Acon.

    trembling of, with, Op.

Eyes, balls of, turned up, with, Œnan.

    black spots before the, with, Glon.

    bright, sparkling, with, Bell., Canth., Coff., Mosch.

    closed, half, with, Cic.

    convulsive, with, Bell., Chin. s., Hyosc.

    dilated, with, Bell., Canth., K. brom., Mosch., Œnan.

    fixed, with, Bell., Cic.

    injected, with, Verat. vir.

    insensible, with, Op.

    rolling, with, Atrop., Cocc.

    staring, with, Hell., Mag. phos., Mosch.

Face, bright red, with, K. brom., Verat. vir.

    cold, with, Bell., Cic., Puls.

    congestion of, with, *Amyl. nit.*, *Arn.*, Atrop., *Bell.*, Gels., Glon., Ign., Œnan., Op., *Stram.*

    convulsive twitching of muscles of,

with, Ant. tart., Bell., Chin. s., Cic.,
Hyd. ac., Hyosc., Lyc., Merc. c.,
Œnan.

Face, distorted, with, Atrop.

expansion of, sensation of, with, Arg.
nit.

expression of deep suffering, with,
Canth.

grimaces, with, Bell.

livid, blue, with, Bell., Cic., Cupr., Glon.,
Hyosc., Lach., Œnan., Verat. a.

œdema of, with, Ars., Canth.

pale, with, Ars., Bell., Canth., Cic.,
Glon., *Ign.*, Puls., Verat. a.

sunken countenance, with, K. phos.

swollen, puffed, with, Canth., Coff.,
Crotal., Glon., Op., Stram., Verat. a.

trembling, spasmodic, of muscles of,
with, Lyc.

twitching of, rapid, with, Œnan.

waxy appearance, with, Ars.

yellowish, with, Canth.

Fainting, with, Cimic., Glon., Lach., Nux
m., Sec., Verat. a.

Fanned, desire to be, with, Carb. v.

Fear of death. See Death.

with, K. brom.

Fear, to be alone, with, K. phos.

Feels strange, Cimic.

Feet, cold, with, Carb. v., Caust., Lach.

Feverishness, with, Caul., Caust.

    absence of, Ign.

Fingers, clinched, with, Cupr., Glon., Mag.
    phos.

    extended and then closed, with, Lyc.

    spread apart, with, Glon.

Flatus, horribly offensive, with, Mosch.

Fright, from, Acon, Op.

    with grief, the exciting cause, Ign.

Frightened appearance before and after,
    with, Stram.

Froth. See Mouth.

Genitals moist, with, Caul.

Grief from fright, the exciting cause, Ign.

Grinning, sardonic, with, Stram.

Groaning, commencing with, Ign.

Hæmorrhage. Consult Repertory on Hæm-
    orrhage.

    with (especially), Hyosc., Sec.

    begins with convulsions after labor;
      every convulsion more blood,
      Hyosc.

    loss of much blood, from, *China*, Crotal.

Hands, cold, with, Carb. v., Caust.

Hands, clenched, with. See under Fingers.

    trembling of the, with, Ars.

    stretched out, with, Sec.

Happiness, foolish, after, Sulph.

Head, bent backward, with, Ign.

    cold sweat on forehead, with, Verat. a.

    congestion of, with, Acon., *Amyl. nit.*,
        Arn., Bell., China, Coff., Glon.,
        Verat. a., *Verat. vir.*

    convulsive motion of, from behind forward, with, *Nux m.*

    dull feeling forehead and vertex, with,
        Gels.

    expansion of, sensation of, with, Arg.
        nit., Gels.

    fulness, sense of, Gels.

    hot, and body cool or natural, with,
        Arn.

    lifting head from pillow, continually,
        with, Stram.

    veins of, distended, with, Chin. s.

Heart, burning distress in region of, constant, with, Verat. vir.

    distress about the, great, with, Hyd.
        ac., Lyc.

    failure, with, Carb. v.

    neuralgic pains about the, with, Cimic.

Heart, palpitation of, with, Glon., K. Phos.,
       Verat. vir.
Heat, or covering up warmly, from., Op.
Hiccough, with, Cic.
Hydrophobia, symptoms of, with, Canth.,
       Hydrophob.
Hysterical, Hyosc., Nux m.
       followed by paralysis, Crotal.
Impressions, very susceptible to, *Cocc.*
Indigestion, from, Nux v.
Injures herself, tries to, Cimic.
Interval between, deep sleep, with grimaces
       or starts and cries, Bell.
       constant motion, tossing about, during,
           Arg. nit.
       convulsive action of face, eyes, etc.,
           during, Chin. s.
       restlessness, great, during, Cupr.
       unconsciousness, during, Bell.
Intestines, great torpor of, with, Nux v.
Irritability, with, Cham., Cocc., Hyosc.,
       Nux v.
Irritation, reflex, from, Chlorof.
Jar, renewed by a, Nux v.
Jaws locked, with, Cic.
       affected, Hyd. ac.
Jerking. See under Muscles and Shocks.

Knee, languor in, great, with, Nux m.

Labor.   Consult conditions, pains, etc., in Repertory on Labor.

     before, Verat. vir.

     ceases and twitching and convulsions begin, Sec.

     commencement of, especially at the, Acon.

     difficult, following, Cocc., Glon.

     during, especially, Bell., Caul., Chlorof., Cinnam., Cupr., Verat. vir.

     during, subject to convulsions, Chlorof.

     during, when attacks begin at periphery and spread centrally, Cupr.

     immediately after, especially, Amyl. nit., Ant. tart., Atrop., Bell., Cic., Cupr., Glon., Verat. vir.

     instrumental, after, Glon.

     pains cease. See Repertory on Labor.

     pains, false, with, Cimic., Nux m.

     pains forcing, violent, with, Sec.

     pains irregular, with, Caul., Cocc., Nux m., Puls., Sec.

     pains severe and tedious, with, Cimic.

     pains spasmodic, with, Cham., Cimic., Cocc., Nux m.

     pains suppressed, from, Op.

Labor, pains very distressing, with, Cham.

    pains weak and ceasing, with, Carb. v., Nux m., Sec.

    pains weak and irregular, with, Caul., Puls.

    protracted, after, Glon.

Larynx, renewal of, from touching the, Canth.

Laughter, convulsive, with, Apis.

    singing, etc., with, Stram.

Left side, commences on the, Lach.

Legs, cramps in the calves of, with, Sec.

    labor-pains tearing down the, with, Cham.

    see, also, Extremities.

Limbs. See Extremities.

Lips, dry, with, Bry.

    blue, with, Cupr.

Loquacity. See Talk.

Mania, especially where, remains after, Verat. vir.

Mental excitement. See Excitability.

Mind, confusion of, with, Gels., Hell., Merc. c.

Motion, better from gentle, K. phos.

    convulsive. See Extremities, Face and Muscles

    in constant, between spasms, Arg. nit.

Motion, loss of, with, Puls.

 renewed by, Cocc.

Mouth, angles of, alternately drawn up and relaxed, with, Lyc.

 foam at, with, Ars., Bell., Cic., Crotal., Glon., Lyc., Nux m., Op., Verat. a.

 foam at, bloody, with, Atrop.

 foam at, may be of a rotten odor, with, Bell.

 opening of the, with, Cupr., Op.

Move, cannot bear to, or to be moved, Bry.

Muscles, alternate extension and contraction of, with, Lyc.

 convulsive motion of, with, Bell., Caust., Hyosc., Op., Plat., Verat. vir.

 fail to act properly, with, Hell.

 prostration and weakness of, with, Gels.

 rigid, with, Amyl. nit., Ars., Cham., Cic., Ip., Merc., Op.

 twitching of, with, Apis, Bell., Cinnam., Gels., Hyosc., Merc. c., Mosch., Verat. vir., Zinc.

 twitching of, between spasms, with, Bell.

 twitching of single, with, Plat.

Nausea, incessant, with, Ip., Œnan.

Neck, drawing in the nape of, with, Hyd. ac.

Neck, worse about the, Lach.

nervous excitement. See Excitability.

Noise or a shock shortens the attack, Hell.

renewed by, Nux v.

Nose, angles of, alternately expanded and contracted, with, Lyc.

Œdema, general, with, Ars.

Œsophagus, constriction of, preceded or followed by, Plat.

Opisthotonos, with, Ars., Cic., Cupr., Ign., Lach., Nux v., Plat., Sec.

Os uteri, hard and thick, with, Gels.

rigid and sensitive, with, *Cham.*, Gels., K. brom.

soft and thick, with, Lob. i.

spasms of, with, Acon., *Caul.*, *Cimic.*

consult Repertory on Labor.

Pain, renewal of, at every, Bell.

labor. See Labor-pains,

Paleness, with. See Face.

Paralysis of left side, symptoms of, Arn.

with, Crotal., Hyosc.

of tongue, right side, with, Bell.

Perspiration, with, Bry., *Stram.*

cold, with, Verat. a., Verat. vir.

hot, with, Op.

sour-smelling, with, Cupr.

Placenta, retained, with, Canth., Sec.

    see Repertory on Retained Placenta.

Presentiment of spasm, she has a, Arg. nit.

Primiparæ, in, Acon.

Prostration.   See Exhaustion.

Proud, haughty spirit, with, Plat.

Pulsations, great, with, Bell., Glon.

Pulse, full, strong, with, Arn., Bry., Gels.,
        Glon., Puls., Verat. vir.

    intermittent, with, Chin. s.

      rapid, very, with, Chin. s., (Pyrog.),
        Verat. vir.

    slow, with, Gels.

    weak, with, Chin. s.

Rage, frequent attacks of blind, biting at
        persons, with, Cupr.

Rapid succession, in, Amyl. nit.

Rash, with, Cupr.

Renewal of.   See the cause of renewal.

Respiration.   See Breathing.

Restlessness, with, Acon., *Arg. nit.*, *Ars.*,
        Bell., Cupr.

    extreme, before, Œnan.

Right side, worse on, Mag. phos.

Rigidity of muscles.   See Muscles.

Saliva, excess of, with, Merc. c., Merc.

Sensibility, loss of, with, Stram., Zinc.

Sensitive to all internal and external impressions, K. phos.

Septic influences, with, Crotal., Pyrog.

Sexual excitement, with, Mosch.

Shivering, shuddering, with, Bell., Cocc., Plat.

Shocks during sleep, with, Cham.

    from head through body, with, Cic., Hell., Hyd. ac.

    or noise shortens the attack, Hell.

    passing through the whole body, conscious of a, before, Laur.

Shrieks, screams, crying out, with, *Amyl. nit.*, Bell., Caust., Cimic., Crotal., *Cupr.*, Hyosc., Lach., Lyc., Merc., *Nux m.*, *Op.*, Stram., *Verat. a.*

Shrinks back from everything on opening the eyes, Stram.

Sighing, with, Caust., Ign.

Sigh, passes off, with a, Cocc.

Singing, praying, etc., with, Stram.

Skin, blueness of, with, Laur.

    cold and blue, with, Hyd. ac.

    hot and dry, with, Acon.

Sleep, loss of, from prolonged, Cocc.

    occurs when she sleeps, none while awake, Lach.

Sleep, see Coma.

Sleepiness, with, Apis, *Nux m.*

> during day, wakeful at night, Merc. c.

Sleeplessness, with, Cimic., Coff., K. brom.

Sobbing, with, Ign.

Sopor. See Coma.

Speech, loss of, with, Bell., Stram.

> stammering, with, Stram.

> thick, with, Gels.

> see, also, Talk.

Spitefulness, with, Cham.

Starts, sudden, with, Bell., Cham., Cocc.

Stiffness of the body and limbs, with, Mag. phos.

Stomach feels as if it would burst with wind, Arg. nit.

> begins with an aura from region of the, Nux v.

Stool, involuntary, with, Arn., Bell.

Strange, feels, Cimic.

Stretching of body backward. See Opisthotonos.

> of body during remission, Atrop.

> of limbs, commences with, Ign.

Stunned, she appears as if. Bell.

Stupid, she feels and looks, Gels.

Stupor, between, Op.

Sudden onset of spasm, Œnan.

Suffocative spells. See Breathing.

Swallowing. See Deglutition.

Sweat. See Perspiration.

Talk, incoherent, with, Cimic., Coff.

Teeth, gnashing of, with, Atrop., Caust., Coff.

Terror, with, Cocc., Stram.

Tetanus, like, tetanic, Cham., Chin. s.

Thirst, with, Acon., Ars., Bry., Caul.

Throat, constriction, sense of tight, with, Crotal.

    gurgling in, on swallowing, with, Cupr.

    worse about the, Lach.

Thumbs, bending in of, with, Atrop., Glon., Mag. phos.

Tongue, bites the, with, Bell., *Cic.*, Œnan.

    paralysis of right side of, with, Bell.

    pushed out and withdrawn, with, Lyc.

Torpor, with, Crotal.

Tossing about, with, Arg. nit., Atrop., Bell.

    about from side to side. See Restlessness.

Touch, renewed by, Nux v., Stram.

    of painful parts, renewed by, Canth.

Trembling, with, Apis, Cocc., Crotal., Lach., Merc. c., Op., Plat.

Twitching of muscles. See Muscles.

Unconsciousness. See Consciousness, loss of.

Uræmia, from, Chlorof., Hyd. ac., Mosch., Œnan.

Urination, desire frequent, with, Canth.
  painful, with, Canth.

Urine, albuminous, with, Apis, Ars., Canth., Chin. s., Crotal., Gels., Glon., Merc. c., Verat. vir.
  clear as water, with, Mosch.
  high-colored, with, Apis, Ars., Canth.
  involuntary, with, Arn., Bell.
  mucus and shreds in, with, Canth.
  profuse, with, Glon., Mosch.
  retention of, with, Hyosc.
  scalding, with, Canth.
  scant, with, Apis, Ars., Canth., Mosch.
  thick as yeast, with, Mosch.

Uterus, inactive, with, Gels.
  see, also, Os Uteri, and Cervix Uteri.

Vertigo, with, Œnan.

Violent spasms, with, Arg. nit., Atrop., Canth., Cham., Cic., Cimic., Lach., Verat. vir.

Vision, dim, with, Gels.

Visions, fearful, with, Bell., Cimic., Stram.

Vomiting, with, Ars., *Cupr.*, Ign., Œnan.

Vulva, moist, with, Caul.

    sensitive, with, Canth., Plat.

    swollen, with, Canth.

Walk about, for relief, must, K. brom.

Warmth, better from, Mag. phos.

    caused by, or covering up warmly, Op.

Water, averse to, Stram.

    sight, sound or drinking, renews spasms,

        Canth., Hydrophob., Stram.

Weakness. See Exhaustion.

Women, broken down constitution of, Cro-

      tal.

    proud, haughty, in, Plat.

    scrawny, poorly nourished, in, Sec.

    weak, in, Cocc., Ign., K. phos.

    consult the other Repertories.

AFTER-PAINS.

Consult other repertories for character-
istics or symptoms pertaining more especially to them, especially that on Labor.

ABDOMEN, bloating of, with the pains a few
      days after labor, Lil. t.

    feels badly in the, Sulph.

    labor-like pains, violent, in, Fer.

    pains felt mostly in, Sep.

Abdomen, pain from, and sacrum, to thighs, Sabi.

> pains run from sacrum to pubes, Sabi.
>
> pains severe, running upward, or upward and backward, Gels.
>
> spasmodic pains in lower, sometimes extending to groins, Caul.
>
> tender, sensitive, to pressure, Cimic., Lil. t., Sabi.

Aching pains, with, Nux v.

Aggravation of pains towards evening, Puls.

> at night, or altogether at, Rhus t.

Air, desires fresh, Cham., Puls.

> averse to, Nux v.

Anus, sensation of a weight in, like a ball, constant, Sep.

> with constant sense of weight in, Sep.

Back, felt mostly in the, Sep.

> bearing-down or forcing in, with, Sep.
>
> with pain in the, Caul., Sep.
>
> with pains in, shooting into gluteal region or hips, K. carb.

Bearing-down feeling, constant, and urging to urinate, Lyc.

> down, strong, with, *Pod.*, Sec., Sep., Ustil.

Bed, least jar of, unbearable, Bell.

Breath, excited by taking a deep, Bry.

Bruised condition of the parts, from, Arn.

Changeable feeling, now better, then worse,
        Puls.

Chest, pain in, with, Caul.

    weak feeling in, with, Stann.

Clots, induced by large, Viburn. op.

Continuous, very severe, pains, Xan.

Contractions are not proper, Cimic.

    intense, but very imperfect, Paris q.

    pain out of proportion to the, Coff.

Covered, desire to be well, Nux v., Rhus t.

    averse to being, Sec.

Cramp-like pains, with, Viburn. op.

Cramps, with terrible, Cupr.

    in the calves, with, Rhus t.

    in the extremities, with, Cupr.

Death, fear of, with, Acon., *Coff.*

Delirium, with, Hyosc.

Delivery, after instrumental, Hyperc.

Despondency, with,

Distant places, pains in, from uterus, Carb. v.

Distressing, very, Cham., Coff., Cupr., Xan.

Endure, she cannot, Cham.

Exhaustion, with, Caul.

Extending from left to right, Con.

Extremities, cramps of the, with, Cupr.

    cramps in the calves, with, Rhus t.

Eyes, balls of, sore and painful to slightest
    motion, Paris q.
    congestion of, with, Bell.
    pain, back of the, Cimic.
Face, fiery-red, with, Fer.
    flushing of, with, Arn., Bell., Cimic.
    sensation as if it were drawn toward the
        root of the nose, then backward, as
        if by a string, Paris q.
Faint spells, weak, with, Sulph.
Fainting after every pain, Nux v.
Feet cold, or very hot, especially the soles,
    Sulph.
Fingers, cramps in, with, Cupr.
Flatulency, with, Pod., Nux m.
Flow. See Lochia.
Forcing pains, Bell., Sec., Sep.
    pains, as if contents of pelvis would be
        forced through the vulva, Bell.
Frantic, rendering her, Cham.
Frequent, one after the other, Rhus t., Sec.
Genitals, very sensitive to touch, Lil. t.
Groins, dragging toward the, Lyc.
    extending to, Caul., Cimic.
    worse in the, Cimic.
Hæmorrhage. See under Lochia, and Rep-
    ertory on Hæmorrhage.

Hæmorrhage, with every pain, of fluid and
   clotted blood, Sabi.
Head, congested, with, Bell.
   severe aching in right side back of orbit,
      with, Cimic.
   severe aching in, Cupr., Fer., Hyosc.,
      Paris q.
   splitting aching, in, Bry., Cimic.
Heat, with, Pod., Sep., Sulph.
Iliac region, with sticking in, from right to
   left, Lyc.
Inguinal region.   See Groin.
Intermitting in multiparæ, Visc. alb.
Irritability, with, Cham., Nux v.
Jar, every, hurts her, Bell.
Jerking and twitching of various parts of
   the body, Hyosc.
Labor, difficult, after, Arn.
   instrumental, after, Hyperc.
   protracted, too, Nux v.
   protracted and exhausting, particularly
      after, Caul.
Light, cannot endure, Bell.
Lips, parched and dry, with, Bry.
Lochia, dark and clotted, Cham.
   discharge feels hot, Bell.
   flow increased with every pain, Bell.,
      Xan.

Lochia, offensive, Nux v., Sec., Xan.
    partly fluid, partly clotted, Fer., Ustil.
    profuse, Cham., Ustil., Xan.
    scant, Nux v., Sulph.
    suppressed, entirely, Paris q.
    thin and brown, Sec.
Loins, labor-like pains in, violent, Fer.
Long-lasting. See Protracted.
Low-spirited. See Melancholy.
Melancholy, with, Cimic., Ign.
Motion, excited by, Bry.
    averse to, Bry., Nux v.
    relief from, Rhus t.
Mouth, dry, with, Bry.
    bad taste in, with, Puls.
Multiparæ, in the, Cupr., *Sec.*, Visc. alb.
Muscular weakness, with, Gels.
Nausea, with, Cimic., Ip.
Nervousness, with, Caul.
Neuralgia, predisposed to, Cimic.
Night, pains worse at, or may have none
    during day, Rhus t.
Noise, cannot endure, Bell.
Nursing child, excited by, *Arn.*, Con.
Painful, very, *Acon.*, Arn., Cimic., *Coff.*, Gels.
    consult Violent.
Pains, a few days after labor, with bloating
    of abdomen, Lil. t.

Pains, distant parts from uterus, in, Carb. v.

    excited by talking, Sulph.

    extending down along genito-crural nerve, Xan.

    extend from right to left, Con.

    feels that she cannot endure the, *Cham.*, Cimic., *Coff.*

    pressing, Sec.

    run upward, or upward and backward, Gels.

    severe, shooting down the thighs, Lac can.

    shooting, K. carb., Lac can.

    stitching, K. carb.

    wants to get away from the, and from herself, Cham.

Piles, bleeding and itching, with, Sulph.

Protracted, prolonged, Acon., Gels., Nux v., Puls., Sec., Ustil., Xan.

    lasting all night, Rhus t.

Pubes, pain from sacrum to, Sabi.

Pulse full, hard, Fer.

Quickly coming and going, Bell.

Quiet. See Motion, averse to.

Rectum, sensation of something in, to be evacuated, Nux v.

Restlessness, with, Cimic., Puls., *Rhus t.*

Restlessness, frequent change of position
   with temporary relief, Rhus t.

Right side, rather worse on, Lac can.

Room, desire to have, warm, Nux v., Rhus t.
   averse to having, warm, Puls.

Sacrum and hips, with severe headache, violent in, Hyperc.
   pains from, around pubes and down
   thighs, Sulph.
   run from, to pubes, Sabi.
   pains severe in, Hyosc., Phos.

Sadness, with, Ign.

Sensitiveness, over, Cimic., Coff., Gels.

Severe.   See Painful.

Shuddering, with, Fer.

Sighing, with, Ign.

Sleep, with half-waking and murmuring, Gels.

Sleepiness, with, Coff.

Sleeplessness, with, Caul., Cimic., Coff., Gels.

Spasmodic pains, especially, Hyosc., Viburn. op.
   pains across lower abdomen, Caul.

Spitefulness, with, Cham.

Sticking in right and left iliac region, with,
   Lyc.

Stool, every pain causes desire for, Nux v.,
   Paris q.

Strong pains, Acon.

Sudden in coming and going, Bell.

Talking fatigues and excites the pains,
       Sulph.

Thighs, pains shooting down the, Lac can.,
       Sulph., Viburn. op., Xan.

Thirst, with, Bry., Cham.
    for large quantities of water, Bry.
    without, Puls.

Throat, dry, with, Bry.

Toes, cramps in the, Cupr.

Trembling, sense of, all over, without actual
       trembling, Sulph. ac.

Twitching and jerking of various parts of
       the body, Hyosc.

Urethra, smarting of, after urination, Lil. t.
    soreness and sensitiveness of, with,
       Hyperc.

Urine, retention of, with, Hyperc., Lyc.
    smarting of urethra after passing, Lil. t.
    teasing to pass, with, Canth., Nux v.
    urging to, with inability to pass, Lyc.

Uterine region, sore feeling in, dislikes to
       move or be disturbed, Nux v.
    neuralgia in and about the, Lil. t.
    very tender, cannot bear weight of cov-
       ering, Lil. t.

Uterus, does not contract properly, Cimic.

    feels as if drawn into a knot, Ustil.

    pains are located especially in the, Sulph.

    pains out of proportion to the contraction of the, Coff.

    spasmodic contraction of the os, Viburn. op.

Vagina, pain shooting upward in, Sep.

Vertigo, with, Fer.

Violent pains, Arn., Cham., Hyperc., Nux v., Paris q., Puls., Viburn. op., Xan.

    consult Painful.

Vomiting, with, Cimic.

Warmth, desire to have, Nux v., Rhus t.

    averse to, Puls., Sec.

Weakness, Caul.

    sense of, and trembling, without actual trembling, Sulph. ac.

Women, elderly, scrawny, who have borne many children, Sec.

    feeble, in, Fer.

    hysterical and nervous, Viburn. op.

    mild, tearful, Puls.

    spare habit, nervous, delicate, Xan.

    consult other Repertories.

THE BABY.

ABDOMEN, hard places in the skin of, and
thighs, quickly increasing, Camph.
deep redness spreading over the whole,
Camph.

Apoplectic symptoms, Acon., Bell.

Asphyxia, Acon., Ant. tart., Arn., Bell.

Breath, anxious, spasmodic, Bell.
gasping for, Ant. tart., Camph., Laur.
jerking, Arn.

Breathless, Acon., Ant. tart., Ars., Laur., Op.

Cyanosis, Lach.

Dead, lies as if, Ars.

Death, apparent, Ant. tart., Camph.

Eyes dilated, Bell.
injected, Bell.
motionless, staring, Bell.

Face, blue, Lach., Laur.
hot, body cold, Arn.
twitching of muscles of, Laur.
very red, Bell.

Features distorted, Ars.

Fever, violent, Camph.

Hot, very, Acon.

Limbs stiff, particularly the knees, Ars.
tremor of, Arn.

Ophthalmia, Acon.

> purulent, Arg. nit.

Paleness, Ant. tart., Ars., Op.

Pulseless, or nearly so, Acon.

Purplish color, Acon.

Skin dry, like parchment, Ars.

Spasmodic rigidity; seems well, but suddenly becomes rigid, etc., Cic.

Spasms, tetanic, bending backward, Camph., Op.

> tetanic, with frightful concussion of the limbs, Ars.

Suffocative form, Ant. tart., Camph.

Swallow, inability to, followed by spasms, Bell.

Syncope, after great loss of blood by the mother, China.

Tetanus, traumatic, Arn.

Throat, rattling of mucus in, Ant. tart.

Trismus, with sudden starting and drawing together of body and limbs, Bell.

Umbilicus open and urine oozing through, Hyosc.

Urine, retained, Acon.

Yellow skin, Acon.

	1	2	3	4	5	6	7	8	9	10	11	12	13	14	15	16	17	18	19	20	21	22	23	24	25	26	27	28	29	30	31	
Jan.	1	2	3	4	5	6	7	8	9	10	11	12	13	14	15	16	17	18	19	20	21	22	23	24	25	26	27	28	…	…	…	**Nov.**
Oct.	8	9	10	11	12	13	14	15	16	17	18	19	20	21	22	23	24	25	26	27	28	29	30	31	1	2	3	4	5	6	7	
Feb.	1	2	3	4	5	6	7	8	9	10	11	12	13	14	15	16	17	18	19	20	21	22	23	24	25	26	27	28	29	30	…	**Dec.**
Nov.	8	9	10	11	12	13	14	15	16	17	18	19	20	21	22	23	24	25	26	27	28	29	30	31	1	2	3	4	5	6	7	
March	1	2	3	4	5	6	7	8	9	10	11	12	13	14	15	16	17	18	19	20	21	22	23	24	25	26	27	28	29	30	31	**Jan.**
Dec.	6	7	8	9	10	11	12	13	14	15	16	17	18	19	20	21	22	23	24	25	26	27	28	29	30	31	1	2	3	4	5	
April	1	2	3	4	5	6	7	8	9	10	11	12	13	14	15	16	17	18	19	20	21	22	23	24	25	26	27	28	29	30	…	**Feb.**
Jan.	6	7	8	9	10	11	12	13	14	15	16	17	18	19	20	21	22	23	24	25	26	27	28	29	30	31	1	2	3	4	…	
May	1	2	3	4	5	6	7	8	9	10	11	12	13	14	15	16	17	18	19	20	21	22	23	24	25	26	27	28	29	30	31	**March.**
Feb.	5	6	7	8	9	10	11	12	13	14	15	16	17	18	19	20	21	22	23	24	25	26	27	28	29	30	31	1	2	3	4	
June	1	2	3	4	5	6	7	8	9	10	11	12	13	14	15	16	17	18	19	20	21	22	23	24	25	26	27	28	29	30	…	**April.**
March	8	9	10	11	12	13	14	15	16	17	18	19	20	21	22	23	24	25	26	27	28	29	30	31	1	2	3	4	5	6	…	
July	1	2	3	4	5	6	7	8	9	10	11	12	13	14	15	16	17	18	19	20	21	22	23	24	25	26	27	28	29	30	31	**May.**
April	7	8	9	10	11	12	13	14	15	16	17	18	19	20	21	22	23	24	25	26	27	28	29	30	31	1	2	3	4	5	6	
Aug.	1	2	3	4	5	6	7	8	9	10	11	12	13	14	15	16	17	18	19	20	21	22	23	24	25	26	27	28	29	30	…	**June.**
May	8	9	10	11	12	13	14	15	16	17	18	19	20	21	22	23	24	25	26	27	28	29	30	31	1	2	3	4	5	6	…	
Sept.	1	2	3	4	5	6	7	8	9	10	11	12	13	14	15	16	17	18	19	20	21	22	23	24	25	26	27	28	29	30	…	**July.**
June	7	8	9	10	11	12	13	14	15	16	17	18	19	20	21	22	23	24	25	26	27	28	29	30	31	1	2	3	4	5	…	
Oct.	1	2	3	4	5	6	7	8	9	10	11	12	13	14	15	16	17	18	19	20	21	22	23	24	25	26	27	28	29	30	31	**Aug.**
July	8	9	10	11	12	13	14	15	16	17	18	19	20	21	22	23	24	25	26	27	28	29	30	31	1	2	3	4	5	6	7	
Nov.	1	2	3	4	5	6	7	8	9	10	11	12	13	14	15	16	17	18	19	20	21	22	23	24	25	26	27	28	29	30	…	**Sept.**
Aug.	8	9	10	11	12	13	14	15	16	17	18	19	20	21	22	23	24	25	26	27	28	29	30	31	1	2	3	4	5	6	…	
Dec.	1	2	3	4	5	6	7	8	9	10	11	12	13	14	15	16	17	18	19	20	21	22	23	24	25	26	27	28	29	30	31	**Oct.**
Sept.	7	8	9	10	11	12	13	14	15	16	17	18	19	20	21	22	23	24	25	26	27	28	29	30	31	1	2	3	4	5	6	

EXPLANATION.—Find in top line the date of menstruation; the figure below will indicate the date when confinement may be ex-pected, i.e. if date of last menstruation is June 1st, confinement may be expected on March 8th, or o[...] [...]er if leap year.

INDEX.

21

PART II.